The Hepatitis C Help Book
Revised Edition

THE Hepatitis C Help Book

Revised Edition

A Groundbreaking Treatment Program
Combining Western and Eastern Medicine
for Maximum Wellness and Healing

MISHA RUTH COHEN, O.M.D., L.Ac.,
and ROBERT G. GISH, M.D., with KALIA DONER

ILLUSTRATIONS by ROBIN MICHALS

ST. MARTIN'S GRIFFIN New York

www.stmartins.com

Library of Congress Cataloging-in-Publication Data

Cohen, Misha Ruth.
    The hepatitis C help book : a groundbreaking treatment program combining Western and Eastern medicine for maximum wellness and healing / Misha Ruth Cohen and Robert G. Gish, with Kalia Doner. — Rev. ed., 1st St. Martin's Griffin ed.
        p. cm.
    Includes bibliographical references.
    ISBN-13: 978-0-312-37272-9
    ISBN-10: 0-312-37272-8
    1. Hepatitis C—Treatment. 2. Hepatitis C—Alternative treatment. 3. Medicine, Chinese.
I. Gish, Robert G. II. Doner, Kalia. III. Title.

RC848.H425G55 2007
616.3'623—dc22

                                                                                    2007005723

First Edition: May 2007

10 9 8 7 6 5 4 3 2 1

A Note to Readers

This book is for informational purposes only. Readers are advised to consult a trained medical professional before acting on any of the information in this book. The fact that a particular therapy, treatment, herb, or supplement is discussed in the book does not mean that it is recommended for every individual. Each person seeking to use the guidelines in this book should be first examined and diagnosed by a qualified health care professional. Similarly, the fact that an organization or Web site is listed in the appendix to the book does not mean that the author or publisher endorses the information they may provide or recommends any of the therapies, treatments, herbs, or supplements they may offer or suggest.

To Ron Duffy and all those with hepatitis C
who have taught us so much
about life, medicine, and
the human spirit

Contents

INTEGRATED TREATMENT PROGRAMS

Acknowledgments

From Misha Ruth Cohen (2006): In the past six years, many more people have learned they have hepatitis C and many more have become infected. And I have met and worked with so many more people with hepatitis C as well as those who want to make this their cause. I want to thank Lorren Sandt, a woman who has become one of my heroes through her tireless work to make HCV a household word and to prevent more people from dying of its deadly complications. Since the last edition, Dr. Gish and I have become members of the Brainstorming Team of the Hepatitis C Caring Ambassadors Program, a group dedicated to helping to educate the public and to help in finding novel therapies and tests for HCV that is managed by Ms. Sandt. I want to thank all the members of the HCCAP Brainstorming Team for helping me to think more broadly and deeply about all aspects of HCV. This edition has again been made possible by Jennifer Weis at St. Martin's Press, who continues to understand the necessity of keeping knowledge about HCV current. I want to thank the countless clients with HCV who I have served at Chicken Soup Chinese Medicine as well as all those who have come to seminars at Quan Yin Healing Arts Center—you have taught me immensely. I want to thank the more than two hundred Chinese medicine practitioners who have attended the Hepatitis C Professional Certification Programs and who go on to share their knowledge in public health settings, educational institutions, and treat people in their practices. I want to thank Carla Wilson, my partner, for standing by me during this intensive process. I especially want to thank Alice Osiecki, Robin Roth, and Cindi Ignatovsky for their countless hours reading, writing, and editing so that this revised edition can be the best possible. And finally, to Kristel McBride, Corrina Rice, Suzanne Stroebe, and all the staff at Chicken Soup Chinese Medicine, who have supported me through keeping the clinic running during this writing process.

Acknowledgments

The Hepatitis C Help Book
Revised Edition

1

Your Best Treatment Options: Combining the Healing Powers of Western and Chinese Medicines

Dear readers,

In the past six years, since we first wrote this book, there have been significant improvements in detection and treatment of hepatitis C. More people are able to stay on their Western medications because we have learned how to reduce the negative side effects, and more and more people are seeing the infection come under control. In addition, there is a growing use of Chinese traditional medicine as complementary therapy for HCV. We are thrilled that to date we have trained more than two hundred Chinese medicine practitioners in the United States, Mexico, and Canada through the Hepatitis C Professional Certification Program.

But as yet there is no universal cure. As the epidemic grows—more than 5 million people are now infected in the United States alone and 40 percent of people with HIV are coinfected with HCV—people with HCV are seeking a deeper understanding of their options using both Western medicine and alternative and adjuvant therapies.

This new, updated edition of *The Hepatitis C Help Book* is designed to bring you the latest information available from both Western and Chinese medicine. We have added a new chapter, The Optimum Interferon Protocol, in order to help people with HCV maximize treatment success. (See chapter 20.)

How did this epidemic sneak up on us? While the infection is not spread casually—transmission occurs only through the transfer of infected blood—more than 300,000 people were exposed through blood transfusions before the disease was first identified in 1989. Thousands more picked it up by sharing intravenous drug paraphernalia, the straws used to snort cocaine, tattooing, and other sources of potential blood-to-blood contact. What makes hepatitis C so frightening from a public health point of view is that those who have the disease seldom realize they're sick when they first become infected. They may remain symptom-free for decades and pass the virus along through shared straws or needles, and even shared toothbrushes and razors.

According to the office of the Surgeon General, the epidemic already costs around $600 million a year. That price tag will skyrocket in the future. More than 80 to 85 percent of those infected will eventually develop chronic liver disease.

The Hepatitis C Help Book is the first guide that offers comprehensive programs that include both Western and traditional Chinese medicine treatments for hepatitis C. The book is designed to inform people who are infected with the virus, as well as healthcare practitioners, about how these two medical systems can be used together to achieve the most effective treatment possible.

Although the two of us come from very different medical traditions and prescribe different medical treatments for hepatitis, over the years we have developed a collaboration. We often refer our patients to one another for diagnosis, Western treatment options, acupuncture, and herbal therapy, knowing that the best care depends on using all available resources for healing.

The Hepatitis C Help Book is a result of our work together and individually. Step by step, we explain how the liver works, exactly what hepatitis C does to the body and how it is diagnosed using Western and Chinese medicine. We outline the full range of treatment options, both Western and Chinese—from drug therapy to herbal formulas, acupuncture to nutritional support, and more.

In addition, we have created self-help programs that promote physical, spiritual, and mental health. You may use them in addition to or separate from your regular Western therapy to help maintain your health and well-being. The programs include:

The Basic Hepatitis C Help Program
Managing Digestive Dysfunction
Dispelling Fatigue
Immune Strengthening
Easing Aches, Pains, Fibromyalgia, and Arthralgias
Addiction Management: Harm Reduction and Withdrawal

We hope these programs will show you new ways to improve the health of your mind/body/spirit.

MISHA RUTH COHEN, O.M.D., L.Ac., and ROBERT G. GISH, M.D.

THE SILENT EPIDEMIC

2

The ABCs (and Beyond) of Hepatitis

It's tough enough having a chronic disease—you are always aware that you are "sick," even when you feel good—but even harder than that for me is how my diagnosis changed the way my family and friends see me. They would deny it, but the truth is they treat me differently than they used to, almost like I was an invalid. I want to shake them and tell them, it's just a virus, not a character trait. *I* am not hepatitis, I *have* hepatitis.

—Larry F., 42, a father of three teenagers, was diagnosed in 1999; he suspects he's had hepatitis C for about twelve years

WHAT IS HEPATITIS?

Hepatitis in all its forms is one of the most common and most devastating diseases in the world, affecting more than half a billion people and costing trillions in health care and lost productivity, not to mention the enormous physical and psychological toll it takes on individuals and families.

Hepatitis is an umbrella term that simply means liver inflammation. A virus may cause it—as is the case with hepatitis C—or it may be caused by an autoimmune response, a chemical toxin, or a drug. Occasionally, hepatitis may unexpectedly develop as a result of infection by some other virus, such as cytomegalovirus, a common complication of HIV.

Some forms of hepatitis cause acute distress, but after a period of weeks or months the infection is vanquished by the body's immune defense system and leaves no lasting negative side effects. Other forms, such as hepatitis C, may fester undetected for years, even decades, and are identified only when severe health problems finally become evident. What unifies all the various types of hepatitis, however, is the cascade of complications that may occur when the inflammation (whatever the cause) leads to extensive scarring of the liver tissue.

Chinese Medicine Notes

In Chinese medicine (CM), unlike Western medicine, no single word, such as hepatitis, is used as a catchall to describe liver inflammations, whatever the cause. Instead, liver disease is viewed in terms of the symptoms it produces and the corresponding syndromes that those symptoms indicate. Each syndrome pinpoints disharmonies that may be affecting Organ Systems and what the Chinese call the Essential Substances—Qi, Xue, Jin-Ye, Jing, and Shen, which give life, power, and emotion to a being.

Furthermore, in CM these syndromes are triggered not by viruses, chemical toxins, or bacteria but by what are called Epidemic Factors and Pernicious Influences.

- The primary trigger of infectious liver disease (such as hepatitis A, B, and C) is the Epidemic Factor Toxic Heat. This form of pestilence is able to affect the healthiest body with great virulence, and it penetrates the body's defenses quickly and easily.
- Once Toxic Heat invades the body, it sets up patterns of disharmony in the Organ Systems and Essential Substances (see page 20 for a detailed explanation of these life-giving essences). These patterns vary from person to person depending on the physical strengths and weaknesses already in the body; for example, someone might have a seasonal allergy and be suffering from Dampness in the Spleen and Lung. When Toxic Heat encounters this condition, it may worsen the Damp condition and trigger fluid retention or diarrhea, both common symptoms associated with hepatitis.
- Toxic Heat also interacts with each individual's basic constitution; for example, someone might be chronically Kidney Deficient, as is almost everyone in America because of diet and lifestyle. When Toxic Heat enters a body that is already Kidney Deficient, it penetrates the Protective Qi and makes a swifter attack on the internal Organ Systems.

Both one's transient disharmonies and basic constitution allow for the development of various disease patterns in association with Toxic Heat. That is why some people progress toward serious complications of one kind, some come down with other types, and still others may not develop them at all. However, as hepatitis C progresses, whatever complications arise, Toxic Heat is always the underlying disease trigger.

In Chinese medicine, in addition to Toxic Heat, six Pernicious Influences—heat, cold, wind, dampness, dryness, and summer heat—are also responsible for disharmonies in the Organ Systems. They can trigger both acute and chronic symptoms of infectious hepatitis.

The syndromes triggered by Toxic Heat and/or Pernicious Influences develop according to the Eight Fundamental Patterns of Disharmony: Interior and Exterior; Deficiency and Excess; Cold and Heat; and Yin and Yang. These terms are used to describe states of disharmony. When coupled with the Pernicious Influences or Epidemic Factors, they form the basis for specific diagnoses; for example, a person with hepatitis C may be diagnosed as suffering from Spleen Qi Deficiency and Damp Heat.

The syndromes that arise from the onslaught of Toxic Heat and/or Pernicious Influences can be used to identify conditions that correspond to various forms of Western hepatitis and hepatitis-related complications.

How You Develop a Disharmony:
The Path of Chinese Medicine Disease Syndromes

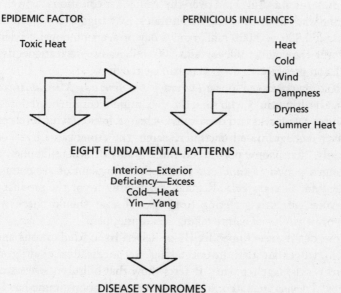

EPIDEMIC FACTOR

Toxic Heat

PERNICIOUS INFLUENCES

Heat
Cold
Wind
Dampness
Dryness
Summer Heat

EIGHT FUNDAMENTAL PATTERNS

Interior—Exterior
Deficiency—Excess
Cold—Heat
Yin—Yang

DISEASE SYNDROMES
OF THE ORGAN SYSTEMS AND ESSENTIAL SUBSTANCES
such as
Damp Heat in the Gallbladder
Spleen Qi Deficiency

ARE ALL FORMS OF HEPATITIS INFECTIOUS?

No. There are five forms of viral hepatitis that are communicable in various ways—some quite easily, others only through the exchange of infected blood. But other forms, such as autoimmune hepatitis and hepatitis triggered by drugs or chemicals, cannot be spread to other people.

Here we will look briefly at these various forms of noncontagious hepatitis. (For in-depth information about medications, chemicals, and herbs that can cause liver inflammation or severely worsen viral hepatitis, see Appendix III, Liver-Toxic Medications and Herbs.)

Poisons—such as alcohol, some prescription or recreational drugs, and environmental pollutants—can cause liver inflammation and may permanently damage the liver. Sometimes toxins can stimulate an autoimmune response, causing the body's disease defense system to go awry and attack the cells in a healthy liver, destroying its ability to function properly.

Alcohol-induced liver damage is the most common form of toxin-produced hepatitis. Because alcohol is metabolized (that is, burned up and cleared from the bloodstream) by the liver, excess amounts—more than two drinks a day—can cause damage. If a person already has hepatitis, drinking any alcohol at all puts a dangerous strain on the liver and vastly increases the risk of developing serious, even life-threatening, complications.

Legal prescription drugs and over-the-counter medications, as well as recreational drugs such as cocaine and barbiturates, may trigger or worsen hepatitis.

More than 2,000 to 3,000 milligrams a day of acetaminophen (Tylenol)—the standard over-the-counter pill contains 500 milligrams—recreational drugs (such as heroin), and prescription drugs can damage the liver.

A 2006 study published in the *Journal of the American Medical Association* reported that healthy adults who took the maximum recommended dose of acetaminophen for two weeks had drastically increased liver enzyme levels that could lead to liver damage. Based on this research, the American Liver Foundation recommends "that people not exceed three grams of acetaminophen a day for any prolonged period of time. . . . This is the equivalent of six 'extra-strength' tablets a day for several weeks. Regular, short-term use of the product is not an issue. Anyone currently suffering from liver disease should check with their physician or hepatologist before taking acetaminophen."

For more details, see Appendix III on Liver-Toxic Medications and Herbs. General guidelines are that anyone taking any medication or drug should be tested for liver damage regularly. If tests show that bilirubin levels are elevated and your ALT levels are 150 or more, stop the medications immediately.[1]

Environmental and industrial toxins such as radiation, solvents, cleaners, and polyvinyl chloride may cause cellular changes in the liver resulting in everything from mild inflammation to cirrhosis, liver failure, and even cancer.

Some herbal remedies may pose a threat. Herbs are potent medicinal remedies, and some may trigger liver inflammation just as a chemical toxin, or an over-the-counter or prescription drug may. In Appendix III, there is an extensive list of those substances that are liver toxic and those that are particularly dangerous for anyone with hepatitis.

WHAT ARE THE DIFFERENT TYPES OF CONTAGIOUS HEPATITIS?

There are five unique hepatitis viruses: A, B, C, D, and E. What was thought to be hepatitis G turns out not to be a hepatitis virus but a GB virus.

Hepatitis A Virus (HAV) is usually contracted through eating food or water tainted with fecal matter. Fruits, vegetables, shellfish, and even ice cubes contaminated by sewage-polluted water can carry HAV. Furthermore, once the virus contaminates a utensil or a piece of food, it remains active for three to four hours. Other routes for the infection to be spread include kissing, oral/anal sex, and any sexual relations that may pose a risk of oral-fecal transmission. Contaminated needles shared between IV drug users are also a possible route. Most infected children generally show no symptoms. As carriers, however, they are infectious for fifteen to fifty days, and during that time they can pass along the virus. Infected adults often experience pronounced symptoms: fatigue, jaundice, fever, nausea, abdominal pain, light stools, and dark urine. In some cases these symptoms can persist up to twelve months. Fully one-third of Americans have evidence of past infection.

There is no specific Western treatment for HAV, other than attempts to relieve the symptoms. However, a person who has close contact with someone who has hepatitis A should receive normal human immunoglobulin (a protein extract from blood; also called "antibody") within two weeks of exposure if they have not been vaccinated against HAV. Hepatitis A vaccine can be given at the same time as the immunoglobulin.[2] Chinese traditional medicine also can be used to ease symptoms and often to shorten the severity and the course of acute distress. There is, however, a highly effective vaccine (using an inactivated A virus) requiring two or three shots for children two to eighteen years old, and one shot followed by a booster six months later for adults. The vaccination is recommended for those traveling in developing countries as well as children living within those high-risk populations, and for anyone who has chronic hepatitis B, hepatitis C, or HIV/AIDS.[3]

Once a person recovers from HAV, he or she is immune. HAV usually produces no serious aftereffects; however, among adults such a severe liver infection can be life-threatening. Even among healthy individuals, one in one thousand cases is fatal, and for those who have HAV and are also infected with HCV and/or HIV, the mortality rate can be as great as 40 percent.

Hepatitis B Virus (HBV) affects more than 2 million people in the United States alone, with 200,000 new cases annually. Experts believe about 5 percent of those people become chronically ill from the disease. In fact, the Centers for Disease Control estimates that currently 1.5 million people have chronic HBV infection and 4,000 to 5,000 people die each year from HBV-related chronic liver disease or liver cancer. Teens and young adults are the most vulnerable, accounting for most of new acute symptomatic cases. Fortunately, the vaccine that is now available is highly effective, and it is the first vaccine ever that can prevent a form of cancer.

HBV is generally an acute disease, lasting less than six months in adults. The infection can cause the liver to become swollen and inflamed, and can trigger fatigue, fever, dark urine, light stools, and jaundice. When it does become chronic, it can cause scarring, cirrhosis, and hepatocellular carcinoma (liver cancer). For children, however, the rate of chronic infection, if HBV is acquired at birth, is more than 90 percent.

HBV is effectively spread through bodily fluids including blood, semen, vaginal secretions, breast milk, and even saliva.[4] The virus can also enter the body through any break in the skin and mucous membranes. Sexual contact may be the most common route of transmission in adults, and the disease is one hundred times more infectious than HIV. Furthermore, the risk is thirty times greater of contracting hepatitis B through a needle stick with a contaminated syringe than contracting hepatitis C through a needle stick. Infants born to infected mothers are also at high risk for contracting hepatitis B. The hepatitis B virus can survive outside the body for up to seven days on a dry surface and is more contagious than HIV (the virus that causes AIDS) and hepatitis C. Currently 1.5 million people have chronic HBV infection and 5,000 people die each year.[5]

Carriers are infectious for an average of eight to twelve weeks. Vaccination (not made with live or attenuated virus) provides protection against HBV for thirteen or more years and is administered in three injections over six to twelve months. It is suggested for all newborns, infants, children eleven to twelve years of age, and any sexually active teenagers. The Hepatitis Foundation encourages parents to vaccinate children within twelve hours after delivery to avoid serious complications if a child is infected and to eradicate HBV entirely. Health-care workers and those who respond to emergency medical situations are also at risk for infection and should be vaccinated. Anyone who has been diagnosed with hepatitis C or HIV/AIDS should also be vaccinated, since infection with hepatitis B can cause severe complications.

Safety concerns about the HBV vaccine have been growing. The CDC states: "Concerns about possible adverse effects of hepatitis B vaccine are being taken seriously, and carefully controlled scientific studies are under way to examine whether vaccination is associated with serious neurological disease in a small number of people. There is no confirmed scientific evidence that hepatitis B vaccine causes chronic illness (including multiple sclerosis, chronic fatigue syndrome, rheumatoid arthritis, optic neuritis, or other autoimmune disorders). Serious adverse events reported after receiving hepatitis B vaccine are very uncommon and may represent coincidence rather than causation. An extremely low rate of anaphylaxis (hives, difficulty breathing, shock) has been observed in vaccine recipients based on reports to the Vaccine Adverse Event Reporting System (VAERS), with an estimated incidence of one in 600,000 vaccine doses distributed. There is no risk of HBV infection from the vaccine. Given the frequency and severity of hepatitis B infection, the benefit of vaccination far outweighs the known and potential risks."

Recent studies indicate that immunologic memory remains intact for at least twenty-three years and confers protection against clinical illness and chronic HBV infection, even though anti-HBs levels might become low or decline below detectable levels.[6]

Any presumed risk of adverse events associated with hepatitis B vaccination must be balanced with the expected 4,000 to 5,000 HBV-related liver disease deaths that would occur without immunization, assuming a 5 percent lifetime risk of HBV infection. Vaccination against hepatitis A is strongly recommended as well for those with chronic hepatitis B.

Hepatitis C Virus (HCV) affects 4 to 5 million people in the United States, more than 2 million people in Canada, and around 170 million people worldwide. The most recent report (in 1996) from the CDC in Atlanta indicates that in the United States 36,000 new cases are reported each year. It is estimated that between 55 and 85 percent of HCV cases become chronic—leading to scarring of the liver and possibly cirrhosis, liver cancer, and liver failure—but many people are unaware that they are infected. In fact, infection with the virus can persist without noticeable symptoms for twenty or more years. HCV is currently the leading cause of liver transplantation in the United States. (Of those infected, 15 to 45 percent do spontaneously recover; however, we do not know how or why.)

Transmission is mainly through exchange of contaminated blood. Blood transfusions used to account for the majority of cases, but that risk has been reduced dramatically. The chance of contracting the virus through blood transfusion in the United States is now less than one in 2 million transfused units of blood. That has decreased due to development of more sophisticated screening tests.

Those most at risk for the disease include people sharing needles or other drug paraphernalia that may be contaminated by blood. Injecting drugs accounts for 60 to 90 percent of all cases. Transmission is also possible through unsterilized tattoo or body-piercing equipment and manicuring tools, such as those used in manicures and pedicures to cut and remove cuticles and calluses. Infection may also happen when inkpots used to store tattooing dyes are contaminated through reflux; this is a potential danger even when tattoo needles are sterile. However, studies show that tattoos, manicures, and pedicures account for less than 3 percent of total HCV infections.

The risk to health-care workers from contaminated needle sticks is 1.8 percent. Transmission occurs between monogamous sexual partners around 3 to 6 percent of the time, and the virus is transmitted from an infected mother to her newborn less than 5 percent of the time. (This number increases to 19 to 27 percent when coinfected with HIV.) Birth risk is 1 to 5 percent.

According to the CDC, the transmission of HCV infection through breast milk has not been documented and is considered likely only if there is bleeding. In the five studies that have evaluated infants born to HCV-infected women, the average rate of infection was 4 percent in both breast-fed and bottle-fed infants.

There is no vaccine for hepatitis C because the virus is unstable, partly due to its genetic structure, and mutates easily. Currently, six different genotypes (clades) of HCV are known and at least thirty different subtypes, each triggering slightly different symptoms and responding differently to available treatments. However, those who have hepatitis C should make sure they receive vaccines against hepatitis A and B, since contracting C along with either of these other viruses can be devastating.

Hepatitis D Virus (HDV), or the hepatitis delta virus, requires the presence of hepatitis B in order to replicate itself. HDV exists only when there is a current infection with HBV. HDV can be acquired at the same time as an HBV infection or as what is called a superinfection, meaning that HDV is acquired after a person already has chronic HBV infection.

HBV-HDV coinfection may lead to more severe disease and can cause a greater risk of fulminant hepatitis (liver failure) than if a person is infected with only HBV. HDV coinfection is usually suspected when a person's condition suddenly worsens and there is a marked increase in the severity of acute HBV symptoms—nausea, fever, jaundice, light stools, and dark urine.

In those rare cases where HBV becomes chronic, if a person gets an HDV superinfection it also becomes chronic. In long-term studies of chronic HBV carriers with HDV superinfection, 70 to 80 percent developed evidence of cirrhosis and other chronic liver diseases—compared with 15 to 30 percent of people with chronic HBV infection alone. Transmitted through the blood, HDV is most frequently found in IV drug users and is less likely to be transmitted sexually than is HBV.

Hepatitis E Virus (HEV) is spread through fecal-contaminated water and food, as is HAV, and its symptoms—always acute and never chronic—are identical to HAV. The main difference between HAV and HEV is that the fatality rate from HEV among pregnant women is 20 percent. The virus can only be identified through laboratory tests. There is no specific treatment, and generally the disease runs its course in a matter of weeks or months. HEV is mostly found in developing nations and rarely in the United States. According to the Australian Hepatitis Council, 1 to 2 percent of those infected can develop sudden and severe liver disease.[7]

Hepatitis G Virus (HGV) is a newly identified virus. Hepatitis G, formerly called GB virus C (GBV-C), is a virus that is related to HCV; however, it is now known that it does not cause hepatitis. The terminology *GB virus C* (GBV-C) is more correct as this virus does not cause hepatitis. Co-infection GBV-C may help people with HIV and improve outcomes.

HGV was found after people who had a blood transfusion developed "post-transfusion hepatitis," which could not be identified as any known virus. It is transmitted by infected blood or blood products and carried in 2 to 5 percent of the U.S. population.

HGV infection can lead to persistent infection for up to nine years in 15 to 30 percent of adults. The long-term outcomes of the infection are not yet known. People with hepatitis A, B, or C can be co- or superinfected with hepatitis G. No vaccine is available for hepatitis G.

Although knowledge is limited about hepatitis G, studies to date show that the hepatitis G virus can cause persistent viraemia lasting for several years. This simply means "presence of virus in the blood" and may not mean the person is sick. However, like any virus, a person with hepatitis G may experience some flu-like symptoms.

No links have been established between HGV infection and chronic liver disease. People with hepatitis G who also have hepatitis A, B, or C do not appear to have worse health outcomes because of the coinfection, and there is little proof that hepatitis G causes serious liver disease.

Vaccination Guidelines for Hepatitis A Vaccine

The Centers for Disease Control (CDC) recommends that the following people be vaccinated:

- people traveling to or working in countries with high or intermediate rates of hepatitis A
- children over two years old in communities that have high rates of hepatitis A or periodic outbreaks. In this country that means American Indian and Native Alaskan populations
- men who have sex with men
- illegal drug users
- people with chronic liver disease, including hepatitis B and C
- workers with an occupational risk for infection
- people with clotting-factor disorders

Although the CDC does not specifically recommend vaccination for those on hemodialysis or with HIV/AIDS, they do say it is safe and effective for those populations. Discuss this with your physician.

Vaccination Guidelines for Hepatitis B Vaccine

The CDC recommends that the following people be vaccinated:

- everyone under eighteen years of age
- anyone older than eighteen who is at risk for the disease—those with multiple sex partners, men who have sex with other men, injection drug users, health-care workers, and anyone who may come into contact with infected blood or bodily fluids

Caution: Do not have the HBV vaccination if you have a life-threatening allergic reaction to brewer's yeast (the yeast used to bake bread).

Balancing the Medical Insights

Western medicine analyzes and treats liver inflammation based on the cause of the inflammation. This allows for research and development of targeted therapies.

Chinese medicine (CM) analyzes and treats liver inflammation and resulting complications based on the symptoms they produce. If viral hepatitis and hepatitis resulting from toxic chemicals both trigger the same symptoms—for example, Damp Heat in the Liver—CM will treat those two cases identically.

Western therapies for viral hepatitis—particularly hepatitis C—often cause negative side effects that make it necessary to stop treatment.

CM therapies are designed to create wholeness and balance from the beginning, so by their very nature they eliminate negative side effects. They may not be able to address all the symptoms of hepatitis, but they rarely create new symptoms.

3

How the Liver Works

> You go along for years without the slightest awareness of what is inside
> you, and then you're told you have hepatitis, and all of a sudden you
> swear you can feel your liver. Take it from me, it's one busy place. Some-
> times I feel like I'm hosting a Grand Prix road race, there is so much ac-
> tivity going on around my poor, overburdened liver.
>
> —MARY S., 52, who contracted hepatitis C from a blood transfusion after the
> birth of her fourth child in 1985

THE LIVER, THE SECOND LARGEST ORGAN (only the skin is larger), is like a
sharp-eyed bouncer guarding the red velvet rope in front of an exclusive night-
club called Your Body: It makes sure the right elements get in and the wrong
ones are eliminated.

The liver enforces its stringent standards for good health using an intricate
network of highly sophisticated cells designed to synthesize, to transform, or to
detoxify nutrients and other chemicals in the blood.

Linked to the digestive tract through a complex system of blood vessels, the
liver takes nutrition from food in the intestines and changes it into essential nutrients such as proteins, fats, and vitamins.

The liver also stores vitamins and sugars (carbohydrates) so the body can have
a ready supply in times of need; and it contains and converts iron and iron-related
molecules into heme, the main oxygen-transporting molecule in red blood cells.
No wonder the immune system, digestive tract, kidney, brain, cardiovascular system, and the regulation of sex hormones are all dependent on a healthy liver.

Understanding how the healthy liver works is essential to understanding what
happens to the body when hepatitis C prevents the liver from doing its job.

BLOOD CIRCULATION AND FILTRATION

The liver has the most complicated network of arteries, veins, and capillaries of
any organ. In fact, a gallon of blood passes through it every 2.6 minutes.

There are two main vessels that transport the blood:

The *portal vein* carries all the blood in the large and small intestines to the liver—and that brings 90 percent of all the nutrition extracted from food in the intestines through the liver's processing plant.

The *hepatic artery*, a branch of a main heart artery called the aorta, brings oxygenated blood from the heart to the liver. Sometimes up to a quarter of all the blood in the body is circulating through the liver.

The portal vein and the hepatic artery are fed by a system of smaller blood conduits that run throughout the liver. These smaller blood conduits in the liver are called sinusoids.

The liver cells, called hepatocytes, are assembled into cordlike structures that are separated by the sinusoids.

These hepatocytes and the sinusoids are contained inside lobules, tiny six-sided structures about one-fifth of an inch wide. Each lobule is dense with blood vessels; a vein runs through its center and is connected to the sinusoids, and six or seven additional blood vessels cluster around each lobule. These vessels include branches of the portal vein (that connects the liver to the digestive tract) and the hepatic artery (that connects it to the heart).

The role of all these blood vessels is to bathe the liver cells with toxins, nutrients, and other chemicals; the liver cells respond appropriately, excreting bile, synthesizing, breaking down, storing, or transporting each element as needed to keep the body healthy and the blood circulating.

In liver disease, scarring of the liver tissue can interfere with the circulation of the blood; this in turn can produce high blood pressure in the portal vein and interfere with the cleansing and nutrition-building functions of the liver.

BILE PRODUCTION AND FAT METABOLISM

One to two quarts of bile—the most important digestive chemical in the body—are synthesized in the liver every day. After you eat a meal, bile made in the liver travels to the major bile ducts and is temporarily stored in the gallbladder until it is needed. When summoned to help with digestion, it travels on through the pancreas and into the intestines, where it breaks down fat molecules so the body can digest them more effectively or excrete them if they are in oversupply.

This process allows the body to absorb the oil-soluble vitamins A, D, K, and E.

Bile helps the body balance cholesterol, 90 percent of which is synthesized in the liver, not derived through the food you eat. Blood levels of this fatty substance—essential for healthy cell membranes and production of sex hormones—can surge in hepatitis C. This happens when bile production is impeded by cirrhosis, or when scarring of the liver reduces the number of active cells available to process cholesterol or makes it difficult for the cells and the blood in the sinusoids to come into contact.

Bile also helps transport the toxins that the liver neutralizes to the kidneys and intestines for excretion.

When bile flow is impaired because of a blocked bile duct (a possible result of gallstones or scar tissue), the whole body is thrown out of kilter: Vitamin synthesis may be reduced, and toxins cleared through the bile may not be excreted from the body. As a result, a person becomes lethargic or depressed, or experiences fuzzy thinking. Jaundice may set in.

The connection between the liver, bile, and feeling down in the dumps has been known for thousands of years. Ancient Greeks coined the word melancholy—it literally means black bile—to describe a state of overall sadness and world weariness. Chinese medicine doctors have long diagnosed Liver Qi Stagnation when a person has similar symptoms: depression and apathy.

BLOOD SUGAR REGULATION

The liver changes glucose (sugar) into glycogen, which it stores until the body needs it to regulate blood sugar levels and to provide energy to the muscles and the brain. In addition, it helps balance amino acids, the building blocks of proteins that are converted into fatty acids and glucose. In Chinese medicine this is associated with the functions of the Spleen Organ System, which encompasses all pancreatic functions.

Changes in blood glucose levels can indicate liver function problems. In fulminant liver failure (that is, sudden liver shutdown) blood sugar levels drop; with cirrhosis, blood sugar levels may skyrocket as a result of increasing insulin resistance and the development of diabetes.

TOXIN REMOVAL

Many toxins such as DDT are lipid soluble; that is, they dissolve in fatty substances, not in water. The liver, using enzymes produced in the liver cells, transforms these fatty toxins circulating in the blood into water-soluble toxins so that they can enter the gastrointestinal and kidney systems and be excreted through the bladder and intestines.

The liver also breaks down natural waste by-products of cell metabolism and other naturally occurring bodily toxins such as ammonia—the by-product of muscle and amino acid metabolism—into less toxic substances (in this case, urea) that can pass through the kidney and become waste.

Bilirubin, a waste product that comes from a breakdown of heme, the central oxygen-carrying molecule in red blood cells, can also act as a toxin. If not cleared out by the liver, this yellowish liquid can produce jaundice, the most vivid symptom of hepatitis and often the first one that alerts a person to the presence of the disease, especially in acute hepatitis or late-stage chronic hepatitis.

The liver also detoxifies drugs, for example, by clearing aspirin from the blood, breaking down alcohol so it can pass from the system, and keeping acetaminophen from being converted to toxic molecules. Excess alcohol harms the liver because it overwhelms the detoxification process, allowing poisons to remain in the liver and damage the tissue.

The liver regulates hormones; hepatitis C disrupts the liver's ability to keep estrogen levels in check. As levels rise in both women and men, complications occur. In men they may include testicular atrophy and breast development.

LIVER ENZYME SYNTHESIS

The liver is awash in enzymes, molecular agitators that are essential for the organ's important work of transforming chemicals and synthesizing nutrients.

AST (aspartate aminotransferase) and ALT (alanine aminotransferase) are liver enzymes used for amino acid metabolism, a process that balances the types of amino acids available for building proteins and then transforms them into proteins. (Tests for AST and ALT enzyme levels are frequently used in diagnosing hepatitis C, despite the fact that they are only crudely indicative of what is going on in the liver: The best use of these tests is to keep tabs on changes in liver inflammation. When ALT or AST levels increase by a factor of ten or more, it can indicate a worsening of the disease.) *Note:* AST used to be called SGOT, and ALT used to be called SGPT; some labs still use that terminology. As of November 2006, standards for normal ALT levels were being reevaluated. The American Association for the Study of Liver Diseases has announced its intention to recalibrate the normal ALT levels from 60 to 30 IU/L to less than 30 IU/L and lower.

Other enzymes made in the liver that are vital to maintaining overall health include alkaline phosphatase and GGT (gamma-glutamyltransferase). Alkaline phosphatase is involved in phosphorus metabolism, which also delivers energy to the body's cells. GGT is used in metabolizing another amino acid, glutamate, which affects tissue oxidation. When fatty deposits cause damage to bile ducts or blockages, these enzyme levels increase. Although the elevated levels aren't necessarily associated with symptoms, blood tests that track these levels can be used to determine the presence and degree of liver inflammation.

PROTEIN METABOLISM

The liver produces and transforms literally thousands of protein molecules a day. Among the most important are fibrinogen, prothrombin, and factors V, VII, IX, and X—proteins that control blood clotting. They are synthesized from amino acids that come from diet, and they are shed in the natural cycle of muscle tissue renewal.

When the liver cannot regulate these proteins, circulatory problems can develop, such as spider veins and hemorrhoids, disorders that may be associated with hepatitis C.

Albumin, another blood protein, is essential to maintain healthy circulation. It acts like a sponge to hold fluid, salt, and water within the blood vessels and may actually help maintain the structural integrity of the vessels themselves. If there is insufficient albumin, as happens when the liver develops cirrhosis, fluid leaks out of the vessels and causes swelling in the ankles and feet.

THE ORGAN SYSTEMS IN CHINESE MEDICINE

To understand how Chinese traditional medicine treats liver disease, it is necessary to take a minute and look at how CM talks about the body's organs in general.

First and most important, Chinese medicine deals with Organ Systems, not the individual anatomical organs that Western medicine has identified. These Organ Systems are responsible for organ functions that are familiar to Western medicine, but they also govern all aspects of the mind/body/spirit. In Chinese medicine there is no separation of the body from the emotional or spiritual aspects of living being.

Some Organ Systems are Yin, meaning they are interior, prone to deficiency and vulnerable to cold; and some are Yang, meaning they are exterior, prone to excess and vulnerable to heat. Together, the Yin and Yang organs create a balanced whole.

Below, each Yin Organ System is paired with the Yang one that complements it.

Yin	Yang
Heart	Small Intestine
Spleen	Stomach
Lungs	Large Intestine
Kidney	Urinary Bladder
Liver	Gallbladder
Pericardium	Triple Burner

You may have noticed in the list above one Organ System that has no correlation in Western medicine: the Triple Burner. This Organ System—which governs metabolism of water in the body by providing a pathway between the kidney, spleen, lungs, small intestine, and bladder—does not exist as a physical entity. It is often called the organ with a name but no shape. This concept is useful in Chinese medicine because all Organ Systems, like much in CM, are defined by their function, not their location. If symptoms arise which indicate that fluid metabolism is disrupted along that pathway, they can be remedied through treatment of the Triple Burner.

Each Organ System is characterized by its interaction with what Chinese medicine calls the Essential Substances and the channels.

Essential Substances

These fluids, essences, and energies that circulate throughout the body nurture the Organ Systems and keep the mind/body/spirit in balance. There are five Essential Substances:

Qi, the Life Force: The presence of Qi is what animates matter, and it is the difference between being alive and being dead. There are at least twelve different types of Qi—some you inherit from your parents and are born with, and some that you acquire through breathing or eating. Every Organ System is governed by Organ Qi. The harmony or disharmony of Organ Qi affects the balance of all Qi in every area of the mind/body/spirit.

Shen, the Mind-Spirit: In Chinese medicine the word Shen is used to encompass the concepts of insight and memory, the act of thinking, and those aspects of a person that are defined as the soul, both ethereal and corporeal. The aspect of the Shen called the Hun, or ethereal soul, is housed in the Liver Organ System.

When Shen is out of balance, it can be treated with medical therapy, just as an upset stomach or a headache would be.

Jing, the Essence that Nurtures Growth and Development: This is infused in the body from one's parents at birth and is depleted throughout life by tension, sickness, and the passage of time.

Xue: Often translated as blood, Xue is not confined to the blood vessels. It also moves through the meridians or channels, and it transports Shen and Qi.

Jin-Ye: This is all the bodily fluids except Xue. It is like rain, essential for life and growth.

Channels

Sometimes called meridians, channels are the great aqueduct system. They extend throughout the body and transport the Essential Substances. Acupuncture stimulates or restrains the flow of the Essential Substances—especially Qi—as they pass through the channels. The acupuncture points where the needles are inserted cause gates along the channels to open or close. The functions of the channels, according to the system of traditional Chinese medicine are as follows:

- to transport Xue and Qi, and regulate Yin and Yang
- to resist pathogens (they are disease-producing agents such as the Pernicious Influences)
- to reflect symptoms and signs of disease and disharmony; the disharmonies that can be read in a channel through acupressure and acupuncture provide a road map to the corresponding disharmonies of Organ Systems
- to transmit the curative force that occurs during acupuncture, which creates sensations such as the spreading of warmth and relaxation through the body, the sense of Qi moving, or a feeling of concentrated heaviness
- to regulate excess and deficiency conditions by transporting Essential Substances throughout the body

In this section we focus on the Liver Organ System, along with the Spleen and Gallbladder Systems, because they are so often affected by hepatitis. However, hepatitis can cause disharmony in all the Organ Systems, as you will see in chapter 5. For a complete description of all the Organ Systems and their associated disharmonies, you can consult Dr. Cohen's book, *The Chinese Way to Healing*.

WHAT THE LIVER ORGAN SYSTEM DOES

In ancient Chinese medicine texts, the Liver Organ System is often called the "general of the army" because it is said to be in charge of maintaining harmony throughout the body. It is also said to function much like the liver in Western medicine—with some added duties:

The Liver Organ System affects digestion, fluid metabolism, and the distribution of energy.

The Liver Organ System controls bile secretion but cannot maintain harmony and the smooth flow of Qi when bile production is disrupted.

It stores and regulates Xue (blood and other substances), which is seen as the mother of Qi—the life force that circulates throughout the body. The Liver

System also removes toxins from the Xue and is responsible for the proper movement of Qi and Xue throughout the body.

It regulates the body by making sure Qi moves smoothly through the channels and Organ Systems.

In addition, it balances emotions—protecting against frustration and sudden anger. Emotional stress disrupts the Liver Organ System and, conversely, liver disease disrupts emotional harmony. In Chinese medicine, the Seven Emotions are joy, anger, sadness, fear, fright, grief, and meditation.

The Liver Organ System also supplies nourishment to the eyes, tendons, and nails.

THE SPLEEN ORGAN SYSTEM—THE LIVER'S PARTNER

As a digestive disorder, hepatitis C primarily affects the Liver and Spleen Organ Systems. To understand the disease in terms of Chinese medicine, you need to know a bit about the Spleen Organ System as well.

The Spleen Organ System creates and controls Xue (as it is involved with the blood in Western medicine). It is also responsible for extracting Qi and fluids from food, transforming these substances into Nutritive Qi and Xue, and, along with the Kidney Organ System, it stores Qi that is acquired by the body after birth.

The Spleen Organ System also maintains the proper movement of ingested fluids and food throughout the body. Qi and the pure fluids are transmitted upward to the Lung and Heart Organ Systems by the Spleen Organ System. Balanced fluid movement lubricates the tissues and joints. This prevents excess Dryness and keeps fluids from pooling or stagnating and creating Dampness. The Spleen Organ System likes Dryness and is affected negatively by Dampness. The Spleen Organ System is also associated with muscle mass and tone, and with keeping the internal organs in place.

THE GALLBLADDER—LIVER'S HELPER

In Chinese medicine the Gallbladder Organ System has a mutually dependent relationship with the Liver Organ System: It stores and secrets the bile that the Liver manufactures. When disharmony strikes the Gallbladder, the Liver is affected, and vice versa. In addition, the Gallbladder Organ System is said to rule the decision-making process—and when the Gallbladder System is not balanced, decisions become impetuous and may be motivated by anger.

Now that we have an overview of both hepatitis and the liver, let's explore the latest insights into hepatitis C and how to diagnose and treat it using both Western and Chinese medicine.

Chinese Medicine Notes

In Western medicine the functions of the liver are to transport and transform nutrients, to help maintain a healthy immune system and digestive tract, to help in the smooth functioning of the kidney, brain, and cardiovascular system, and to regulate sex hormones. In Chinese medicine these functions are understood as being the result of the harmonious collaboration of several different Organ Systems.

- For example, while the Liver Organ System regulates the Qi and Xue (the life force and blood) and harmonizes the emotions, the Spleen Organ System affects fluid metabolism, energy levels, and transportation and transformation of Nutritive Qi—the life energy that comes from food.
- The Kidney Organ System is responsible for the underlying body energy, sexual function, elimination of bodily fluids, clear thinking, and the will. When there is fluid retention, as often happens in advanced liver disease, or fuzzy thinking—another side effect—the Kidney Organ System is involved. People who fight off hepatitis generally have strong constitutions, and that's often associated with a strong Kidney system. The amount of Kidney energy you have is associated with how much Qi (life force) as well as Jing (essence) you have in your body when you come into this world.
- The Heart Organ System may reflect Shen disturbances that are strongly associated with liver disease. It may also reflect Xue (blood) Deficiency, insomnia or nervousness, which often accompany a chronic illness.

Body Basics: How the Liver Works

In Western medicine the liver functions as the gatekeeper and regulator of nutritional health and as a purifying system.

The liver weighs about three pounds and contains four sections, or lobes.

Within the lobe, lobules contain liver cells and passageways for blood circulation, called sinusoids. It is within the lobules that the specialized liver cells transform chemical substances into nutrients the body can use, or neutralizes potential toxins to protect the body from damage.

Nutrition and toxins from the digestive tract are transported to the liver via the bloodstream through the portal vein.

The hepatic artery brings oxygen-rich blood from the heart to the liver.

Because the liver plays a major role in the circulation and the composition of blood, its health has an impact on all body systems, from hormone regulation to thinking.

Balancing the Medical Insights

In both Western and Chinese medicine the liver is a central repository and regulator of the blood. It is instrumental in digestion and nutrition, and when it is not functioning optimally, every other system in the body—from the thyroid to the kidney—can be affected.

Chinese medicine, as distinct from Western medicine, also focuses on the liver's relationship to emotional health. (Remember, the Liver Organ System houses the ethereal soul, one part of the Shen or mind-spirit.)

Many symptoms associated with hepatitis are not treated as separate disorders in Western medicine. In Chinese medicine, however, every syndrome that appears can be treated by working to restore harmony to affected Organ Systems and Essential Substances.

Western medicine provides analysis of the liver's biochemical functions in ways that Chinese traditional medicine cannot.

4

Getting Hip to Hepatitis C

After I was first diagnosed about eight years ago, I felt pretty good for about three or four years. Then suddenly things became worse. I was dizzy, disoriented, and had piercing pain. But my viral load was low, and doctors kept telling me that a lot of people with a load of half a million didn't have symptoms like mine. It made me feel like I had a pretty extreme case somehow. Hard to figure out. I felt awful. They put me on antidepressants, which I stopped taking after a day or two. I couldn't stand what they did to me. Finally, the doctors figured out I had a hiatal hernia. My viral load continues to go up and down—sometimes it's around 100,000; sometimes it's more than double that. But I got the hernia treated, and I'm feeling a whole lot better. They wanted me to start interferon, but I'm glad I didn't. Maybe I will later, or they will come up with a better treatment. For now, my advice if you feel really bad is to persist; make the doctors figure out what is going on. Sometimes it is a combination of hepatitis C and some other physical problem. If everyone is focusing on hepatitis C, other problems may be missed, and you may suffer unnecessarily.

—JUDY S., 48, a marketing executive

THE BEST PROTECTION AGAINST HCV and its complications is to know how it is transmitted, to recognize the signs of infection and symptoms of the disease, and to eliminate or reduce the risk factors.

During the early phases of hepatitis C infection, people may innocently spread the disease to others who are then equally unaware that they have the disease. They in turn can spread it, and so on and so on, until we face a public health crisis of enormous proportions. The lifetime health care costs for the more than 5 million Americans infected, excluding liver transplants, will be more than $400 billion.[1] Tomorrow the costs will be even higher. "Although the incidence of acute hepatitis C has declined, there is a large reservoir of chronically infected Americans who can serve as a source of transmission to others and who are at risk of the severe consequences of chronic liver disease . . ." warns the CDC.

HOW IS HCV SPREAD?

HCV is spread through blood. A small segment of those with HCV contracted it through contaminated blood transfusions, hemodialysis, or blood products received before 1992 when a careful screening process was begun. Many of these people are just becoming aware of their infection or are developing serious symptoms of the disease. We will be dealing with the repercussions of these previous infections for years to come, even as the population in danger of new infections is changing: Today in the United States around 60 percent of people who contract HCV are IV drug users sharing contaminated needles.

There have been reports of a small risk of infection through monogamous sexual activity with an infected partner and from mother to newborn child, but these may depend on undetected blood exchanges as well. What is more, according to the CDC, about 10 percent of those with HCV don't know how they contracted the virus.

The most common routes of infection are as follows:

- shared IV drug needles. The HCV virus can live outside the body (on a surface at room temperature) for anywhere from sixteen hours to four days, and it is not easily killed with chlorine bleach, which does kill HIV rather dependably.
- the use of nonsterilized instruments for tattooing, acupuncture, and body piercing
- shared cocaine snorting straws. Minuscule droplets of blood from the nasal passage are deposited on the straws and then spread to the next user.
- shared personal grooming items such as razors, toothbrushes, scissors, and manicuring equipment, which may carry blood residue.
- unprotected sex. The virus is present in the menstrual blood of infected women, so sexual intercourse at this time creates a potentially hazardous situation. There have been reports of transmission of HCV through sexual intercourse outside menses and between males, but there is current debate as to whether this is actually possible without the presence of a skin or tissue tear or some other disease that provides an opening in the skin of both the infected person and the potential recipient. Whatever the reason, the CDC reports that high-risk sex—identified as sex with multiple partners and/or between males—increases the risk of transmission by as much as 20 percent.

According to an overview of current data on HCV from the American Academy of Pediatrics Committee on Infectious Diseases, published in the March 1998 issue of *Pediatrics,* "Among sexual partners of persons with chronic HCV infection who apparently have no other risk factors for infection, the average prevalence of anti-HCV, that is, antibodies to the HCV virus in the blood, indicating previous exposure was 5 percent (range, 0 to 15 percent). Two studies have found a higher anti-HCV prevalence among the female partners of positive men compared with the male partners of positive women."

And a study reported in 1997 in the *Journal of Infection*, in an article entitled "Absence of Hepatitis C Virus Transmission but Frequent Transmission of HIV-1 from Sexual Contact with Doubly Infected Individuals," concluded that in heterosexual couples—who have not been studied as much as homosexual couples—40 percent of those with no other possible route of infection became HIV positive during the course of their relationship, while 52 percent who were IV drug users became HIV positive. At the same time, no cases of HCV infection were detected in the thirty people whose only risk exposure was heterosexual sex with their partner; however, 95 percent of drug users became HCV positive.

According to the CDC, there is no evidence that the virus is spread through oral sex.

- transfusions of contaminated blood. This risk factor has sharply decreased, however. Testing of the blood supply for HCV began in 1990; a standardized test became available in July 1992. Prior to 1990, tainted donor blood was one of the most common routes of infection. In the early 1970s the risk of contracting some form of hepatitis from a unit of blood was around 1 in 20. Now the risk of contracting HCV from a unit of blood is less than 1 in 3,300; the risk for hepatitis B is 1 in 250,000. In the United States, transfusions with tainted donor blood account for less than one in every 2 million transfused units according to the CDC.

CAN I GET HEPATITIS C FROM A TOILET SEAT? . . . AND OTHER UNNECESSARY WORRIES

HCV is not present in bodily fluids such as urine, saliva, or semen unless they contain blood particles. HCV is not spread through the air; you cannot catch the virus if an infected person sneezes or coughs near you. Close contact such as hugging cannot spread the virus, either. Researchers are not certain, however, whether a mother can pass the infection on to an infant through breast milk. If it is possible, the chances are less than 2 percent unless the mother's nipples are cracked or bleeding, presenting a serious transmission risk. According to several studies and the American Medical Association, mothers who are coinfected with HIV experience transmission rates of HCV to their newborns of around 17 percent.

WHO SHOULD BE TESTED?

- Anyone who has ever received a blood transfusion, hemodialysis, organ or tissue transplant prior to 1992.
- Anyone (such as hemophiliacs) who received blood clotting factor concentrates produced before 1987.
- Anyone who has had intimate contact with or lived with someone infected with HCV.
- Anyone who has ever injected street drugs, even if it happened only once.
- Anyone with a history of body piercing or tattooing.
- Anyone with a history of multiple sex partners and/or sexually transmitted disease.
- Healthcare, emergency medical, and public safety workers who have experienced needle sticks, cuts, or mucosal exposure.
- Anyone who suspects he or she has had the general symptoms of hepatitis such as feelings of nausea, depression, or lethargy, especially when accompanied by dark urine or light stools.
- Newborns or infants of HCV-infected mothers.
- Anyone with persistently high AST and ALT liver enzyme levels.

Remember, a regular blood test will not determine whether or not you have been infected. Your doctor must request blood tests for liver enzyme levels and for viral forms of hepatitis (HAV, HBV, HCV).

DOES HCV EVER JUST GO AWAY?

Fifteen percent (or less) of all people who contract HCV will have a self-limited case in which their immune system defeats the virus, according to L. B. Seeff, M.D., senior scientist (hepatitis C) at the National Institutes of Diabetes and Digestive and Kidney Diseases in Bethesda, Maryland. Dr. Seeff reported this in July 1998 on the *Journal of the American Medical Association* Web site. Who they will be and why it happens is unknown. Chinese medicine surmises that those with strong Qi and Jing may be able to fight off infection more effectively.

Chronic HCV infection develops in 75 to 85 percent of those infected. Among that group, 20 percent develop cirrhosis over a period of twenty to thirty years, and at least 5 percent will die of liver disease—that is, according to CDC, between eight thousand and ten thousand people a year in the United States. The true figure is probably higher, as testing for HCV is not prevalent.

WHY ISN'T THERE A VACCINE FOR HCV?

Unlike the viruses that produce hepatitis A and B, the hepatitis C virus is very unstable. It mutates often, evading the protective antibodies in a person's immune system that might be produced by a vaccine. In addition, there are six genotypes (or clades) of HCV (the result of viral mutations) found in different populations around the world. These genotypes respond to Western drug treatment differently and produce slightly different disease patterns.

These days it is important to have your genotype identified so your doctor can tailor your Western medicine treatment to it. People with genotype 1 should be given therapy for one year. Those with genotype 2 should talk to their doctors about the possibility of receiving six to twelve months' treatment. Recent studies indicate that combination therapy can result in sustained virologic response (SVR) of up to 85 percent of those with non-1 genotypes and 25 to 50 percent of genotypes 1a and 1b.

Genotype 1: Subtype 1a is found most often in the United States, the United Kingdom, and Europe. Subtype 1b is found mostly in Japan and Europe. These genotype subsets are the least responsive to Western medical treatments with interferon and ribavirin. Currently, subtypes 1a and 1b account for 65 to 75 percent of chronic HCV in the United States.

Genotype 2: Subtypes 2a, 2b, 2c, and 2d are found mostly in Japan and China.

Genotype 3: Subtypes 3a, 3b, 3c, 3d, 3e, and 3f are found mostly in Scotland and other parts of the United Kingdom.

Genotype 4: Subtypes 4a, 4b, 4c, 4d, 4e, 4f, 4g, 4h, 4i, and 4j are found mostly in the Middle East and Africa.

Genotype 5: Subtype 5a is found mostly in Canada and South Africa.

Genotype 6: Subtype 6a is found mostly in Hong Kong and Macau.

IS THERE A CURE?

There is no certain cure for HCV, but some Western treatments reduce the viral load to undetectable levels, keep those levels low, and act as liver-protecting agents. This is interpreted by some as a "cure," since years after treatment the most sensitive tests cannot find any trace of the virus in the blood or liver. While this does not mean that the virus has been completely eliminated from the body—it may lurk in tissue and organs where it cannot be measured—it does offer some hope that permanent suppression of virus replication is a realistic goal.

In China there is a long history of effective treatment for liver disease, but the approach is very different from Western drug therapy. Many of the herbal remedies are able to protect the liver from the damage of viral inflammation, even though they do not reduce the viral load. In addition, there are antiviral herbs that appear to hold the virus in check. The combination of these two therapies can produce an effective treatment and protect the quality of life without causing any harmful side effects, although it is not a cure in the Western sense of the word.

WHAT WESTERN TREATMENTS ARE AVAILABLE AND DO THEY WORK?

There are only two approved drug therapies for HCV at this time—interferon and ribavirin—although researchers are exploring several interesting potential treatments. (For more detail, see chapter 7.) Interferon and ribavirin are effective long-term for about 50 percent of cases and may cause severe side effects.

WHO SHOULD BE TREATED?

Western doctors initiate treatment with interferon or a combination of interferon and ribavirin when a person has antibodies to HCV, a measurable viral load and elevated AST and ALT liver enzyme levels, and has had a liver biopsy that reveals evidence of chronic hepatitis that is progressing. People with severe symptoms, regardless of their test results, or a rare condition called cryoglobulinemia, are also good candidates for treatment.

However, not everyone with HCV is a candidate for drug treatment. Therapy is not generally recommended outside of controlled trials for patients who have:

- clinically decompensated cirrhosis (cirrhosis that has progressed toward imminent liver failure) because of hepatitis C
- normal aminotransferase levels (ALT less than thirty independent units per milliliter)
- received a kidney or heart transplant, which present an absolute contraindication because treatment will increase risk of rejection. Liver transplant recipients may be considered on a case-by-case basis. Dr. Gish advises that you consider having treatment within a clinical research study and that you make sure your doctor is a specialist in interferon and transplant
- liver cancer

- women (and men) planning to conceive a child, or any pregnant woman
- specific contraindications to therapy, such as severe psychiatric disease or coronary artery disease.

For more detail on treatment options and obstacles, see chapter 7.

WHAT ARE THE SYMPTOMS OF HCV?

It is difficult to offer a neat list of HCV symptoms, because only 30 to 40 percent of those who contract the disease have any symptoms at the time of initial infection. Furthermore, according to the National Institutes of Health Consensus Statement on HCV, the course of the disease is affected by the various characteristics of the many genotypes and subtypes of the hepatitis C virus itself, by geography, alcohol use, coinfection with other viruses, and other unexplained factors.

Initial Symptoms: When first infected, 10 to 20 percent of people experience nonspecific symptoms such as malaise, abdominal pain, fatigue, and loss of appetite. Around 5 percent have jaundice, which in a way is very positive, since it increases the chances for prompt diagnosis and treatment. Other symptoms that can emerge during the initial period of infection include fuzzy thinking, depression, and digestive problems. Rarely is there any severe liver distress during the initial period. Only 15 percent of people require hospitalization when they are first infected, but occasionally the infection triggers fulminate hepatic failure, which is life-threatening. This is most likely to affect those who are immunodeficient or have a preexisting liver disease.

Of those infected, 80 percent develop antibodies to HCV within fifteen weeks of exposure, and 97 percent by six months. After six months of infection, if the immune system has not cleared the virus from the blood, the disease is considered chronic.

Chronic HCV-Related Symptoms: Noticeable symptoms caused by the virus itself, not by associated complications of the disease, can come and go depending on the strength of the infection at any given time, a person's life stresses, and the presence of other viral infections. However, over the course of the disease, 85 percent of people will experience intermittent symptoms such as fatigue, depression, short-term memory problems, digestive upset, joint and muscle pain, and headaches. Sometimes these are severe enough to interfere with quality of life; sometimes they cause barely a ripple. Elevated liver enzyme levels, a symptom of liver cell injury, are present in two-thirds of those infected, but fully one-third show no evidence of elevated levels at all (using current testing reference values).

Over time, the virus infiltrates the portal tracts (the portal vein and associated blood vessels) and hepatocytes (the basic liver cells), causing local death of liver cells. As the disease progresses, the inflammation causes scarring (fibrosis) in the portal tracts and the tissue cells that help maintain liver function (parenchyma). Contained in these areas, the fibrosis remains mild and the symptoms are generally minor. If the inflammation causes the fibrosis to spread between the portal tracts, it can lead to cirrhosis, a degenerative condition that causes increasing destruction of liver cells and interferes with normal liver function.

Once cirrhosis develops, symptoms of more advanced liver disease may include depression, chronic fatigue, disturbance of blood glucose levels, trouble with digestion, nutritional deficiencies, fluid imbalance, swelling, and more. Advanced HCV can also trigger non-liver-related disorders such as arthritis and kidney disease, which cause joint pain, fever, and fluid retention.

It is important to remember that there is no correlation between the level of viral load and symptoms. Some people with relatively low viral loads have very troubling symptoms, while some with high loads are symptom-free. There is also no absolute correlation between liver enzyme levels and the amount of liver damage sustained, which is why, although you need to have these measures taken, for diagnosis of level of liver damage nothing is as definitive as a liver biopsy.

WHAT DOES "VIRAL LOAD" MEAN AND WHAT LEVELS ARE CONSIDERED GOOD?

In order to confirm that a person is actually infected with HCV after testing positive for HCV antibodies, an HCV viral load test is performed to confirm infection. This test is necessary because up to 45 percent of people exposed to HCV clear the virus through natural immune response, but they still have antibodies.

Also, viral load measurement can help predict how well HCV drug treatment will work. The lower the HCV viral load before interferon treatment, the more likely it is that a person will respond to current HCV therapies.

Viral load tells you how many International Units (IU)—"copies"—of the virus exist in one milliliter of your blood. This correlates with "infectious units" and potentially the number of infectious viruses in a drop of blood. To determine viral load, a PCR (polymerase chain reaction) test may be used during the initial diagnostic process and again during interferon treatment to see if the person's immune system has vanquished the disease. The bDNA test (branched chain DNA assay) can be used to measure viral loads between two thousand and 50 million copies. And the even more sensitive test, TMA (transcription mediated amplification), can measure viral loads as low as five copies per milliliter.

HCV VIRAL LOAD TESTS

Qualitative Viral Load Tests

This type of test tells us whether or not there is any HCV RNA in the blood, but it does not tell us the quantity. If HCV is detected, a positive result is reported; if HCV is not detected, the test result is negative. People who test positive for antibody and negative for virus should be tested at least twice by a qualitative test such as the TMA or the ultrasensitive PCR test. Quantitative tests, as discussed below, can be used as well for this purpose. If the quantitative viral load test is negative, this means that a person has cleared the virus and implies a cure of infection, whether through interferon treatment or through natural immune responses.

Quantitative Viral Load Tests

These tests measure the quantity of the virus in your blood. They are often used to see which drug treatment should be used. If interferon treatment is already in progress, these tests can help determine if the virus is being cleared and the treatment is working.

Three Types of HCV Viral Load Tests

- **PCR** (Polymerase chain reaction)—PCR tests measure HCV RNA in the blood to tell if there is an active infection. These tests can measure small amounts of virus (10 to 50 IU/mL).
- **bDNA** (Branched-chain DNA)—The bDNA test only measures medium to high viral loads (>500 IU/mL). This means that if a person has a viral load below 500 IU/mL, this test may not be able to detect the virus.
- **TMA** (Transcription-mediated amplification)—The TMA test allows for the building blocks of genetic material, like RNA (called nucleic acids), to be detected in the blood. This test can measure very small amounts of virus (as few as 5 to 10 IU/mL). This test is used both to determine initially if a person who is has HCV antibody actually has HCV or during treatment to test if HCV has been cleared from the body

INTERPRETING VIRAL LOAD TEST RESULTS

The HCV viral load is often reported as low or high.

The most common way that a doctor tells a person with HCV about viral load is IU/mL (International Units per milliliter), formally known as copies/mL (copies per milliliter). The conversion from copies to IU is usually a factor of 5.

When expressed as copies/mL:

- Low: less than 2 million copies
- High: more than 2 million copies

When expressed as International Units (IU/mL):

- Low: less than 800,000 IU/mL
- High: more than 800,000 IU/mL

There is no standard conversion formula for converting the amount of HCV RNA reported in International Units (IU/mL) to copies per milliliter (copies/mL). The conversion factor ranges from about one to about five HCV RNA copies per IU. Most lab reports will list the conversion from IU/mL to copies/mL used by that specific lab.

Viral load test results may vary depending on how a blood sample is handled and stored. Also, results may vary from lab to lab. Therefore, most HCV experts suggest that people with HCV have viral load testing done by the same laboratory each time and using the same test, since many laboratories have multiple assays.

If a viral load test finds no HCV RNA, a person's viral load is said to be undetectable. Whether viral load is reported as undetectable depends on which test is used. PCR and TMA tests can measure viral loads much lower than those a bDNA test can detect. It is possible that the blood of an individual with a very low viral load (even by TMA measurements) may still contain HCV. Although extremely unlikely, it is possible that the virus may not have been truly eradicated from the body.

Please note that in some lab reports, changes in viral load are also expressed in logs. A log change is a tenfold increase or decrease. This is a unit 10 value, thus a value of 7.6 logs would be slightly greater than 10 million IU per mL. A one log drop in viral load is measured by decreasing the number by one zero. For example, a one log drop in a viral load of 10,000,000 IU is 1,000,000 IU; a two log drop in a viral load of 10,000,000 IU is 100,000 IU.

Viral load test results have many uses, including confirmation of HCV infection, as well as predicting and measuring drug treatment response before, during, and after interferon therapy. Quantity of virus in the blood has not been correlated with the risk of sexual transmission.

There is no evidence that there is any relationship between HCV viral load and disease progression or severity of disease except in patients who have undergone liver transplantation. Some people and physicians become confused by this fact, since this is different for HCV than HBV and HIV. In HBV and HIV, viral load is directly correlated to severity of disease and risk of disease progression.

A significant decrease in viral load while on drug therapy indicates that treatment is working. If a TMA or another very sensitive qualitative test does not detect the virus, a person is considered to have a complete virologic response if on treatment.

If at four weeks on treatment a person with HCV tests undetectable by TMA or another very sensitive qualitative viral load test, she or he is considered to have a rapid viral response (RVR) and has a 97 percent chance of ultimately clearing the virus permanently at the end of the course of treatment.

At the twelve-week point of anti–HCV drug treatment, a 2-log drop in viral load or elimination of detectable HCV indicates that the medications are working and is defined as an early virological response (EVR). There is a 68 to 83 percent chance, depending on genotype and other factors, that this person will permanently clear virus (cure) if he or she completes the full course of interferon therapy.

If a person does not achieve a 2-log drop in viral load or elimination of detectable HCV after twelve weeks, it is unlikely that he or she will be able to eradicate HCV from his or her body at the end of forty-eight weeks of treatment. Some people are now being treated for seventy-two weeks, especially if they have a slow viral response or, more important, have not had a RVR early in treatment. However, the treating practitioners should monitor each person according to his or her own profile in order to determine how long the drug treatment should be given.

Viral load measurements are also used after drug therapy ends to monitor for relapse—that is, to see if the virus becomes detectable again after being undetectable when treatment was completed. Typically, a person who undergoes interferon treatment and tests undetectable at the end of treatment is again tested at six months after the end of treatment. If the test is again undetectable, especially by TMA or another very sensitive qualitative viral load test, a person is considered to have a sustained viral response (SVR).

WHAT ARE THE COMPLICATIONS OF HCV?

There are many complications of HCV, not only because of its long course but because it disrupts the functioning of so many important bodily functions and processes. Out of one hundred people with HCV, twenty will develop cirrhosis, which can lead to many other devastating disorders and diseases. Five of one hundred will develop primary liver cancer. In fact, hepatitis C is currently the leading cause of liver transplantation in the United States, accounting for between one-fourth and one-third of all liver transplants. That is why prompt attention to your diet and lifestyle and appropriate treatment is so important. Luckily, if you are careful and monitor yourself over time, you can do a great deal to maintain your quality of life and your health. On the other hand, if you are reckless and put extra strain on your liver—for example, by eating too many fats—you increase your risk of developing life-compromising and life-threatening complications. For detailed information on complications and treatment suggestions, see chapters 6 and 7.

IF I HAVE HCV, AM I AT GREATER RISK FOR GETTING OTHER FORMS OF HEPATITIS?

The risk of contracting other forms of viral hepatitis is not inherently greater because you have hepatitis C. However, if you are using recreational drugs, having sex with multiple partners, or participating in activities that expose you to the risk factors associated with those other hepatitis infections, you are at risk.

The risk of developing noninfectious toxic hepatitis is increased because liver sensitivity is greater once you have chronic liver inflammation. Those who have HCV need to be particularly careful about taking substances that are liver toxic, or combining drugs that cause added liver damage. For details, see chapter 3.

IF I HAVE HIV, SHOULD I BE WORRIED ABOUT HCV?

Yes. Up to 40 percent of those infected with HIV also have HCV, and the combination makes HCV much more damaging to the liver much more quickly than without the coinfection. Furthermore, fully 20 percent of people with HIV who also have HCV produce no antibodies to the hepatitis virus, and a simple blood test does not reveal the infection. Therefore, everyone who is HIV positive should have a blood test to check for HCV antibodies. If the results are negative and liver disease is still suspected, you should then receive a PCR test (a viral load test) to make sure you aren't one of those who have the infection without producing antibodies.

Once you are diagnosed with HCV, treatment choices are difficult and must be carefully considered, since medications for HIV and HCV can interact negatively. For more information on coinfections see chapter 6.

WHAT CAN I DO TO TREAT MYSELF?

Chronic HCV responds very positively to many lifestyle changes that you may choose to make.

Altering your diet so that it is low in fat (around 20 percent of calorie intake a day), high in vegetable proteins, and low in simple sugars and animal protein can do a great deal to spare the liver. (See chapter 9 for more detail.)

Abstaining from all alcohol and recreational drugs is also a very positive step. Intake of even small amounts of liquor—a third of an ounce a day—may increase progression of the disease for those with chronic HCV, whether or not they have developed cirrhosis.

In addition, a whole variety of stress-reduction techniques including Qi Gong and meditation (see chapter 11) can strengthen the immune system and lessen the burden on the liver.

The use of other Chinese, Western, and natural therapies can be beneficial, but if you are considering self-prescribing any herbs, patent medicines, or medicinal substances, *don't*. Not only are some substances liver toxic, but they may interact with your other medications. It is important that you always consult with your doctor and Chinese medicine practitioner or other qualified licensed health-care practitioner before taking any supplement or natural remedy on your own, as there are always new reports and new studies being performed.

Self-care is essential and will go a long way to improving your health and the quality of your life, but it should not be done without consultation with your Chinese medicine practitioner and Western physician.

MAY I HAVE ALCOHOL?

Drinking alcohol is the single worst thing you can do to your liver. Those who persist in drinking after diagnosis for HCV increase their risk of developing severe cirrhosis and a long list of very unpleasant associated disorders. This dramatically increases the risk of developing liver cancer. Furthermore, liver transplants often are denied to people who continue to drink alcohol after they've been diagnosed with hepatitis.

DO I HAVE TO TAKE WESTERN DRUGS?

You are in control of your care, and clearly no one can make you take any treatment that you don't want. Treatment decisions must be based on a careful evaluation of the risks and benefits to you. Collect as much information as you can about every treatment option you are considering and then make an informed decision. You may choose to use only Western therapies. You may consider combining Western and Chinese therapy. You may rely on Western diagnostic tests and use only Chinese treatments. Or you may use only Chinese medicine.

HOW DOES HCV AFFECT EMOTIONS AND LIBIDO?

In Western medicine it is the responsibility of the liver to maintain a proper chemical balance within the body. In addition to duties such as regulating cholesterol, producing bile for food digestion, and providing clotting maintenance for the blood system, the liver is responsible for regulating hormones, storing vitamins, and producing proteins and energy. When these functions come under assault, the biochemical system that reacts to and triggers emotional responses is thrown out of balance. Add to that the stress, anxiety, and worry that can plague a person who is diagnosed with a chronic infectious disease, and you have created an emotionally volatile environment.

SEXUAL DESIRE

Fully felt and expressed sexual desire relies on a rather delicate balance of hormones. If hepatitis C interferes with the liver's ability to regulate hormones, the libido will suffer. Men can develop elevated estrogen levels that cause them to lose sexual function, and women may find they suffer erratic hormone levels that cause severe PMS-like symptoms, which are never particularly conducive to romance. In addition, sexual activity takes energy, and the kind of weary fatigue that can accompany a chronic viral infection may make a person too tired to be interested in sexual activity. This can lead to frustration and depression.

Couples may need to explore new ways of relating sexually or of maintaining a feeling of intimacy and closeness during times of sexual abstinence. Professional counseling is always an option in this type of situation.

We also know that the loss of libido can be a side effect of interferon treatment, but stress and exhaustion generally appear to be the primary culprits in any chronic illness.

STRESS RESPONSE

Corticosteroids are a family of adrenal hormones released into the bloodstream in response to a perceived threat or stressful situation. Sustained high levels of cortisol in the blood are thought to contribute to the development of many maladies including depression, drug addiction, hypertension, diabetes, cancer, multiple sclerosis, and stroke. In addition, cortisol is an immunosuppressant, which can decrease a body's ability to battle HCV. This can create a situation in which stress causes proliferation of the symptoms of HCV, which in turn causes stress and suppression of the immune systems that worsen the results of HCV infection, and on and on.

During times of acute excitement or stress, other hormones such as adrenaline are also released into the body. If the liver has difficulty processing these hormones, a sustained period of excitement can produce feelings of fatigue and trigger flare-ups of HCV symptoms such as nausea. To lessen these potential problems it is important to make sure you get enough sleep, eat well, and, if possible, practice stress-reducing techniques such as Qi Gong, yoga, or meditation.

DEPRESSION AND HCV

Chronic depression can result from the stress and the biochemical changes triggered by HCV. Unfortunately, it is not always taken seriously or recognized as a symptom of HCV, but it is a very real medical fact that doctors need to address if they are to combat this disease expeditiously. It is not uncommon to find that people who have been under treatment for depression for many years are infected with HCV. HCV was only discovered in 1989, and up until then, and unfortunately to this day, many doctors treated the emotional symptoms of HCV as something "all in the head." Herbal antidepressants, such as St. John's Wort, and prescription antidepressants, such as Paxil, are safe to take if needed. Acupuncture can also be used to ease depression.

HCV Positive? Take Care

If you have hepatitis C, you want to be vigilant about protecting others from infection. Here are some guidelines:

- Don't donate blood, body organs, other tissue, or semen.
- Don't share personal items that can be contaminated with blood, such as toothbrushes, any dental products, manicure or pedicure equipment, or razors.
- Cover cuts and skin lesions to keep from spreading infectious blood or secretions.
- Don't use or inject street drugs; if you do inject drugs, obtain treatment to stop and prevent relapse.

If you are injecting drugs, take these precautions:

- Never reuse or share syringes, water, or drug preparation equipment.
- Use only new sterile syringes to prepare and inject drugs.
- Obtain syringes from a reliable source so you know they are new and clean.
- Use fresh tap or sterile water to prepare drugs.
- Use a new or disinfected container ("cooker") and a new filter ("cotton") to prepare drugs.
- Clean the injection site with a new alcohol swab prior to injection.
- Safely dispose of syringes after one use.
- If you get a tattoo, insist that the ink and ink container be unused and unopened. Reflux into the bottle can pass on the disease.

Tips on Preventing Sexual Transmission

Sexual transmission of HCV is a relatively rare event for those who are not coinfected with HIV. For monogamous heterosexual couples who only have vaginal intercourse, the risk appears slim to none. However, there are some convincing reports that men who have sex with men (MSM), with many sexual partners, and who engage in high-risk behavior are at increased risk for acquiring HCV infection. Also, people with sexually transmitted diseases (STDs) such as gonorrhea, chlamydia, and syphilis, or people with HIV and HBV may be more likely to transmit HCV to their partners. In order to transmit HCV from one person to another there must be blood-to-blood contact involved in the high-risk behavior. Epidemiological studies suggest that the transmission rate among individuals who engage in high-risk behavior may be as high as 25 percent.

For a person with HCV who has a steady partner and who does not engage in high-risk behavior, there are no recommendations for changes in sexual practices. Both partners should make any decision about using barriers for sexual practices. Although there is no evidence of sexual transmission during the menses, it may be prudent to abstain from sexual intercourse or use barrier precautions during the menstrual cycle. Consideration should also be given to testing exposed sexual partners for antibodies to HCV, and if positive, evaluating them for the presence or development of chronic liver disease.

For persons with multiple partners or who engage in high-risk behaviors that could include blood exposures, safer sex practices are strongly recommended to protect their partners from HCV and themselves from acquiring sexually transmitted diseases. STDs can complicate hepatitis C and cause serious health problems themselves. Recommendations include abstinence, reducing the number of partners, informing all prospective partners about any HCV infection, and using latex condoms. Although no study has confirmed the effectiveness of latex condoms in preventing infection with HCV, based on data from HIV and other diseases, it has been determined that they may reduce transmission.

Who Is HCV Positive?

Having antibodies to the hepatitis C virus in your blood is an indication that you once had or currently have the infection. It is estimated that 15 to 45 percent of people who become infected overcome the disease completely, but they will carry the antibodies for many years. According to the Centers for Disease Control:

- The highest rates of HCV antibodies are found among injection drug users and hemophilia patients—60 to 90 percent of them are HCV positive.
- Moderate rates—20 percent—are in hemodialysis patients.
- Lower rates—1 to 10 percent—are present among persons with a history of blood transfusion before 1990, of high-risk sexual behaviors, or of sexual or household exposure to persons with chronic HCV infection.
- Health-care workers have a very low incidence of infection—1 to 2 percent.

Chinese Medicine Notes

There has been only limited study of the effect of traditional Chinese medicine treatments on viral hepatitis in the United States, but the Chinese have done many studies on the effects of herbs on viral infection and the immune system. Although these studies often were not done under double blind or well-controlled circumstances, or reported only the positive results, they do provide useful insights and information when read carefully. An extensive list of studies on the effects of herbal formulas on liver function and liver disease is given in Background Sources, in the back of the book.

Chinese Medicine Notes

According to traditional Chinese medicine, the onset of viral hepatitis is generally associated with what are called excess Damp Heat or Damp Cold syndromes.

Damp Heat may be characterized by jaundice, nausea, fever, and pain along the side of the torso; Damp Cold may be characterized by decreased appetite, abdominal pain, and feeling cold while having a fever.

Chronic hepatitis is often associated with a continuance of acute syndromes plus a syndrome such as Liver Qi Stagnation or Spleen Qi Deficiency. Liver Qi Stagnation may be characterized by elevated liver enzymes, a swollen liver and spleen, and fatigue; Spleen Qi Deficiency may be characterized by fatigue, nausea, muscle weakness, and loose stools.

Advanced chronic viral hepatitis with severe cirrhosis and other complications is associated with the development of the patterns of Xue Deficiency and Xue Stagnation. Xue Deficiency may be characterized by a shrunken liver and, often, normal liver enzyme levels. Xue Stagnation may be characterized by stabbing pain along the side of the torso and an abdomen that hurts with movement.

Chinese Medicine Notes

If you adopt the philosophy of Chinese medicine as your guiding light, you will be able to create a program for healing based on the unity of the mind/body/spirit and on the importance of self-care and preventive treatment. Chinese medicine offers a way of thinking about managing chronic illness that can dramatically improve your quality of life and help you get the most out of whatever particular treatments you decide to pursue in consultation with your physician and practitioner.

Balancing the Medical Insights

Understanding hepatitis C—in fact, the discovery of the virus that causes it—is very recent in the West. The treatment of the symptoms and Chinese syndromes involved in hepatitis is very ancient in China.

Western medicine's understanding of hepatitis C is based on laboratory tests that measure viral load, enzyme levels, and other markers of the disease. Doctors now make quantitative assessments of the progression of the disease and try to tailor treatment to the degree of liver destruction.

Chinese medicine in the twenty-first century uses the lab-based information as a guide and a check on its long-established techniques for diagnosis and treatment.

5

Diagnosis East and West

In many ways I think becoming sick with hepatitis C has improved the quality of my life. I take such better care of myself; I eat better, I exercise regularly, I meditate and have reduced unnecessary negative stress. And through various support groups I have met the most remarkable people, people I would never have met otherwise. Of course I wish I wasn't ill, but I have to tell you, it has also had its rewards.

—JEFF F., 57, while on his second round of
interferon therapy and using acupuncture

WESTERN MEDICINE USES LABORATORY-BASED TESTS to diagnose HCV. Some tests detect the presence of HCV antibodies, elevated liver enzymes, and the virus itself in the bloodstream. Others assess the amount of cell damage the virus has caused to the liver.

Traditional Chinese medicine, if practiced separately from Western medicine, diagnoses chronic infectious liver disease by studying its symptoms in all their various manifestations, from complaints about depression or sluggish digestion to the color and coating on the tongue. In addition, the symptoms associated with hepatitis C involve many different Organ Systems. The Spleen, Gallbladder, Kidney, Triple Burner, and Heart Organ Systems, in addition to the Liver Organ System, are all commonly understood to be sites of disharmonies related to infectious liver disease. That is why, when diagnosing disorders associated with hepatitis C, a traditional Chinese medicine practitioner may identify Spleen Dampness or Kidney Yin Deficiency as the source of symptoms.

Chinese medicine's reliance on symptoms and signs to form a diagnosis of disharmony means that, unlike Western medicine, it can hone in on subtle emerging disturbances in Organ Systems long before overt and serious liver dysfunction sets in and long before the viral infection has been diagnosed via laboratory tests.

This chapter offers a look at both the Western and Chinese approaches to diagnoses. The goal is to help you understand what your Eastern or Western medicine practitioner is telling you about your level of disease progression. The more information you have, the more confident you can be about the treatment choices you make. However, the suggested programs do not separate the two approaches: Diagnoses and treatment for HCV use a combination of Eastern and Western thought and techniques. The strengths of each offer people with HCV the best chance to maintain a high quality of life throughout the long course of the infection.

WHAT ARE THE LAB TESTS FOR HEPATITIS C?

The available tests for detecting HCV fall into six categories:

1. *A blood test that indicates if liver enzyme levels are elevated.* This is often the first clue to possible liver disease. Elevated liver enzymes indicate that there is inflammation in the liver. The enzymes are released into the bloodstream when a liver cell is damaged, becomes ruptured, and dies. But levels don't give you solid information about the cause or the degree of the damage. In fact, determining enzyme levels at any one point in time is not as important as tracking large swings in enzyme levels over time. You may have early liver inflammation with little or no sign of elevated enzymes, or you may have advanced cirrhosis and low enzyme readings. Only during the initial phase of major liver cell injury do enzyme levels spike dramatically. At that point they provide a more accurate reflection of the degree and progress of the disease, particularly when compared to previously lower levels.

    Nonetheless, you will probably hear a lot about AST (aspartate aminotransferase) and ALT (alanine aminotransferase) levels. You are well advised to avoid comparing your readings with others who have HCV or worrying about moderately fluctuating levels; moderate is defined as a change that is less than a fivefold increase or decrease. Also, 30 percent of the time, people with chronic hepatitis C have normal AST and/or ALT levels according to the average laboratory reference ranges.

    Tests for other liver enzyme levels, such as GGT and alkaline phosphatase, can also indicate liver damage. But it is best to rely on a liver biopsy to confirm that the disease is active and progressing. In very late stages of liver disease, so-called synthetic tests that measure the liver's ability to synthesize proteins and other substances are the standard means of evaluation.

2. *A blood test called ELISA II looks for the presence of antibodies to the virus.* If the results come back positive for HCV, physicians confirm the finding with a PCR test. This is necessary because ELISA II can determine that exposure to HCV happened but it cannot confirm if the infection is current or occurred in the past and is now eliminated from the body.

3. *A PCR (polymerase chain reaction) assay measures the viral load in your blood-stream by targeting the RNA within the virus.* This test will determine if the virus is active and multiplying in the bloodstream.

There are two drawbacks to the PCR test:

- Results can vary from lab to lab. Some labs claim they can find as few as five to ten viral particles per milliliter of blood, but others are far less precise.
- From week to week your viral load may fluctuate wildly, increasing or decreasing by a factor of ten. And even more dramatic fluctuations can happen if you drink alcohol or if there are changes in your immune system—say, for example, you get the flu.
- The PCR test rarely (less than 2 percent of the time) produces a false positive—indicating that you have HCV when in fact you do not. However, around 5 percent of the time the test will register a false negative, missing an active infection that is producing viral load levels too low to register. Repeated PCRs or more sensitive tests may be necessary to get a clearer picture.

4. *A blood test to determine exactly which genotype of the HCV virus you have.* This is important because, as discussed earlier, various genotypes react differently to medications, and knowing the genotype allows the doctor to determine the optimal length of treatment with combination therapy of interferon and ribavirin. (HCV subtypes 1a and 1b are relatively resistant to interferon and to combination therapy. Subtypes 2 and 3 are much more likely to respond positively.)

5. *Imaging tests such as a CT scan or ultrasound.* These are used to get a clearer picture of your liver's size, any structural changes that might have happened as a result of inflammation, and the condition of the portal vein and hepatic artery. The CT scan can also be used to identify early liver tumors. People with cirrhosis may rely on a series of ultrasound tests instead of repeated X rays to determine if liver cancer is developing.

6. *A liver biopsy to allow the doctor to discover the degree of liver damage and the stage of the disease.* Of particular interest is whether or not cirrhosis has developed. A biopsy can also:

- clarify other test results that may not be conclusive;
- alert the doctor to the need to begin treatment with Western medications (if advanced fibrosis/cirrhosis has been discovered);
- determine if the person has any liver disease resulting from medications;
- assist the doctor in establishing a cancer screening schedule if cirrhosis is revealed.

A biopsy removes a small amount of liver tissue—usually less than 1/5,000th of the liver. The tissue is then examined under a microscope to see what cell damage has occurred. Although the results are generally accurate, about 5 percent of the time the biopsy underestimates the amount of inflammation or scar tissue, and less than 1 percent of the time it leads to an overestimation of damage. Biopsies are often done every three to five years to keep track of the disease's progress or to monitor responses to antiviral medication or traditional Chinese medicine. The gold standard is for the treating physician to do the biopsy instead of referring the patient out for the procedure, and that biopsy is done with the concurrent use of sonar imaging.

The risks associated with a biopsy include these:

- bleeding (one in five hundred patients)
- a blood transfusion or further surgery (one in two thousand patients) because of excessive bleeding
- puncturing the lung, gallbladder, kidney, or intestine (one in three thousand patients)
- pain (one in five patients)
- death (less than one in ten thousand patients)

RESULTING DIAGNOSIS: THE STAGES OF HEPATITIS C

Doctors can determine the stage of your HCV infection once they have the results of your liver biopsy. Identifying the stage helps them determine treatment options, but it doesn't reveal much about how long you've had the disease or how long until you progress to the next stage. The time line is quite particular and unpredictable for each individual.

Stage I indicates minimal scarring of the liver. This stage used to be called Chronic Persistent Hepatitis C or Mild Chronic Active Hepatitis C.

Stage II means that scarring has developed and extends outside the portal tracts—the areas in the liver that house the blood vessels and are the first areas affected by liver inflammation.

Stage III means that the fibrosis is spreading or bridging out slightly to adjacent portal tracts.

Stage IV means that the fibrosis has progressed into cirrhosis and advanced scarring of the liver tissue. Often simply referred to as cirrhosis, in this stage many of the complications associated with HCV develop.

WHAT OTHER LAB TESTS MIGHT MY DOCTOR RECOMMEND?

Once your doctor has diagnosed the stage of HCV infection, she will monitor you for development of complications using several blood tests that pinpoint changes in liver function, including:

- a test for levels of bilirubin, the substance that triggers jaundice. Rising levels indicate that the liver is no longer able to process this naturally occurring by-product of red blood cells' life cycle.
- a test for alkaline phosphatase (similar to the GGT or gamma-glutamyl transferase test) that measures liver enzyme levels and also indicates liver inflammation and damage
- a test for serum albumin that can reveal if the liver's ability to manufacture or process vital nutrients is deteriorating or if a person's nutritional habits are poor
- a test for clotting factors that checks prothrombin (PT) time and levels and evaluates the overall clotting function of at least five clotting factors
- a test for platelet levels, which can help determine whether the spleen is destroying platelets—a possible sign of cirrhosis

WHAT SORT OF PHYSICAL EXAM SHOULD MY WESTERN DOCTOR PERFORM?

The art of diagnosis depends as much on intuition and ingrained knowledge as it does on the results of blood tests and biopsies. But these less quantifiable processes are not as formally recognized in the Western medical tradition as they are in traditional Chinese medicine. How much a physician relies on perception and personal examination for diagnosis varies widely. Nonetheless, any physician who suspects or knows that you have liver disease should conduct a physical exam that includes the following steps:

- Evaluate the patient's cardiovascular health—looking for signs of hypertension or hypotension, rapid heartbeat, inflammation, and redness of the palms.
- Check for signs of jaundice of the skin and scleral icterus, or yellow eyes. This condition can indicate a build-up of bilirubin in the blood system and can be a warning sign of hepatitis.
- Perform a complete abdominal exam, including feeling the liver to assess size and texture, and checking for fluid accumulation in the torso, hands, and feet.
- Check for neurological status, including mental clarity, memory, hand flapping, or asterixis and sleep disorders.

- Look for broken veins called spider veins on the chest and face, which are an indication of cirrhosis.
- Notice if a person has a sweet smell or *fetor hepatiticus* on his or her breath.

WHEN DO I START TREATMENT WITH WESTERN MEDICINE?

Treatment with Western drug therapy has been linked to lab test results and the development of complications. Many physicians recommend that anyone with elevated liver enzymes, the development of fibrosis, or a diagnosis of early cirrhosis is a good candidate for antiviral drug therapy. While advanced (decompensated) cirrhosis or liver cancer may decrease the possibility of antiviral drug therapy, some doctors will offer it under very close supervision. Symptoms such as severe fatigue and joint aches, systemic disease such as cryoglobulinemia, or even a patient's concern about being infectious (a rare event) may also lead to treatment.

Recent studies, however, have indicated that early and aggressive use of antiviral therapy (interferon and ribavirin), even before much damage or any symptoms have occurred, may slow disease progress and may offer the best chance for clearing the virus from the blood (or at least lowering it to undetectable levels). Exactly when this therapy should be initiated is an individual decision made by the doctor and the person with HCV.

- *Start self-care immediately*. It is vital that self-care be initiated immediately upon diagnosis. Lifestyle changes are essential, including adjustments to diet, stress reduction, regular moderate exercise, elimination of recreational drugs and all alcohol, making sure you get sufficient sleep, and careful monitoring of possible liver-toxic properties of any over-the-counter or prescription drugs taken for other conditions. For details about how to get started in these areas, see chapters 9 and 11.
- *Chinese medicine treatments can begin with the first appearance of symptoms or disharmony*. As explained below, the use of herbal therapy, acupuncture, Qi Gong exercise, meditation, and other natural healing techniques may be initiated at the first sign of subtle shifts in the body's balance and harmony. A Chinese medicine practitioner may pick up indications of liver inflammation even before a formal diagnosis of infection with HCV is advanced. Treatment can begin immediately upon such diagnosis.

HOW A CHINESE MEDICINE DOCTOR DIAGNOSES HEPATITIS C

Diagnosis depends on a practitioner's powers of observation. There are no lab tests. Instead, using what are called the Four Examinations, a Chinese medicine doctor looks for signs and symptoms of disharmony in the mind/body/spirit.

The goal of the Four Examinations is to determine what type of disharmony the Essential Substances (Qi, Xue, Jing, Jin-Ye, and Shen), Organ Systems, and/or channels are experiencing and which of the Eight Fundamental Patterns of Disharmony (Cold, Heat, Interior, Exterior, Deficiency, Excess, Yin, and Yang) are involved.

Sometimes a practitioner goes through the Four Examinations step by step, but many times the experienced doctor uses them as an informal guide to help shape intuition and casual observation.

The Four Examinations

The heart of the diagnostic process, the Four Examinations, relies on inquiring, looking, listening/smelling (these two seemingly different acts are grouped together; in Chinese they are the same word), and touching.

Inquiring: By asking you questions about yourself the practitioner learns about your mind/body/spirit. You reveal a lot about your well-being through the information you provide in response to specific questions and through your tone of voice, your emotional expression, and your body language. The questions will focus on:

- your reaction to heat and cold
- your patterns of perspiration
- if and when you experience headaches or dizziness
- the type of pain you may have
- your bowel and bladder functions
- your thirst, appetite, and taste
- your sleep patterns
- your sexual functioning, sexual activity, and reproductive history
- your general medical history
- your general physical activity
- your emotions

Looking: Looking is focused on an examination of your tongue, facial color, and body language.

The tongue's color, moisture, size, coating, and location of abnormalities reflect the body's inner condition. They indicate your state of health in general, and also correspond to specific organ functions and disharmonies, particularly in the digestive system. This makes it a powerful diagnostic tool in understanding Organ System disharmonies. However, the tongue's appearance is just one part of a larger picture that is assembled from the Four Examinations.

Facial color provides another clue as to the nature and severity of any disorder or disharmony. Chinese medicine states that five colors appear on the face: red, green, yellow, white, and black. A healthy face generally has one predominant color, but several may be visible. Miriam Lee, L.Ac., from Palo Alto, California, has refined the characterizations of facial colors as follows:

- *Red* is associated with the Heart Organ System and Xue. If the face is a fresh red, the Xue is Hot. If the face is dark red, the Xue is Stagnant. If it is light red, the Xue is Deficient.
- *Green* is associated with the Liver Organ System and circulation of the Xue. If veins on the face appear green-purple, the Xue is Hot. If the veins appear green-black, the Xue is Stagnant. If the condition is severe, the veins appear black.
- *Yellow* is associated with the Spleen Organ System. If the face appears light yellow, the Spleen Organ System is Damp. If the face appears deep yellow, Heat has accumulated. If it is dark yellow, Heat is the result of Xue Stagnation. Withered yellow indicates a Heat Deficiency.
- *White* is associated with the Lung Organ System, which regulates Qi and breathing. If exhalation is insufficient, the face becomes gray-white in color. If inhalation is inadequate, the face appears pale and lusterless.
- *Black* is associated with the Kidney Organ System. If the face is cold and black, the Kidney Organ System is not filtering Xue properly. If the face color is black but bright and moist, the condition can be treated. If the face is not shining, the condition is not good. If the black is withered, the Kidney Organ System's Yin is dry. If the face is cloudy and dark, the Kidney Organ System's Yang is dying.
- When there is more than one color present, as is often the case with HCV when the Liver, Spleen, and sometimes the Kidney Organ Systems are involved, the diagnostic process is further refined.

Body language provides the practitioner with the third set of diagnostic clues gathered through looking, as follows:

- A heavy-footed walk, loud voice, and sloppy, spread-out posture may point to Excess patterns of disharmony.
- Frailty or weakness, poor posture, and a shy receding nature can indicate the presence of a disharmony associated with Deficiency.
- Fast, jerky, impulsive movement and an outgoing personality indicate disharmonies associated with Heat. If also associated with a full red face, high energy, and a loud voice, then both Heat and Excess may be at work.
- Cold patterns of disharmony are associated with slow and ponderous but

not sloppy movements and a pale face. When linked with a low voice, shortness of breath, or passivity, Cold and Deficiency may be at work.

Listening/Smelling: These two observational techniques can tell a practitioner a lot about a person's basic constitution and about the patterns of disharmony that are making the person ill.

Listening focuses on a person's tone of voice, breathing patterns and the sound of coughing to diagnose patterns of disharmony:

- A loud, strident voice indicates an Excess pattern of disharmony, as does the sudden onset of a violent cough.
- A weak, low voice that doesn't project and a weak cough indicate Deficiency.

Losing your voice or hoarseness can indicate either Deficiency or Excess. Wheezing arises from Dampness.

A person's smell can also tell the practitioner a lot about the kind of internal disharmonies that are at work:

- A strong stench from secretions or excretions indicates Excess and Heat.
- A weaker odor indicates Deficiency and Cold.
- A sweet, fetid odor, called fetor hepaticus, is associated with Spleen Organ System disorders.

Touching: Touching involves evaluating a person's pulse and assessing his or her response to the application of pressure at specific points.

Pulse reading is a difficult and subtle art that demands intense training and concentration. Unlike lab tests that return results a week or so later, the pulse gives us an immediate snapshot of what is going on in the body. It reveals Qi's energetics and fluid levels of Xue, Jing, and Jin-Ye, and in some systems of acupuncture it reveals the health of the channels.

There are twenty-eight pulse qualities that a practitioner looks for. The most common are floating, slippery, choppy, wiry, tight, slow, rapid, thin, big, empty, and full.

A disharmony in the pulse can indicate that an Essential Substance such as Qi or Xue is out of balance. It can pinpoint disorders of the Organ Systems and reveal the patterns of the disorders, such as Dampness or Heat. For example, a wiry pulse has a rhythm like a taut guitar string—strong and responsive but without any undulation. It may indicate that the Liver Organ System has Stagnant Qi. However, there are no absolute meanings to pulses. They contribute to diagnosis only when viewed in context with other diagnostic techniques.

Sensitivity to touch, feelings of pain, or absence of sensation when the acupuncture points along the channels are palpated is an indication that there is disharmony in the channels and the associated Organ Systems.

Pain that is not confined to a specific location indicates Stagnant Qi.

Pain in a specific area or point may indicate Stagnant Xue.

Pain that is eased by the application of pressure is due to Deficiency.

Pain that feels worse with pressure is due to Excess.

Pain that feels better with warmth is associated with Cold.

WHAT ARE THE RESULTS OF ALL THIS ASKING AND LOOKING AND LISTENING AND SMELLING AND TOUCHING?

Once an examination is completed, if your practitioner suspects you have infectious liver disease, she should send you to a Western doctor for lab tests to confirm the diagnosis. The practitioner will also have arrived at a Chinese medicine diagnosis for your complaints and will set out a proposed course of treatment that may include acupuncture, herbal formulas, dietary guidelines, and Qi Gong meditation and exercise.

WHAT ARE THE CM DIAGNOSES ASSOCIATED WITH HEPATITIS C?

If you have hepatitis C, you will probably be diagnosed with one or more causes of disharmony and associated syndromes. Toxic Heat is the primary disease trigger. Known as an Epidemic Factor, it creates the initial flu-like symptoms that some people experience when first infected with HCV, as well as those symptoms that plague many people intermittently for years: nausea, fatigue, itchy skin, and a nagging sensation that something toxic is present in the body.

Toxic Heat is also responsible for the cascade disharmonies in the Liver, Spleen, Gallbladder, Kidney, Heart, and other Organ Systems that contribute to the major complications associated with HCV. (For detailed information on complications, see chapter 6.)

When Toxic Heat disrupts Spleen and Liver Organ System functions, the body can no longer properly transform food into energy and transform fluid into Qi and Xue. Symptoms include loose stools, bloating, gas and flatulence, and/or dull pain in the abdomen, needing to take naps after meals, and frequent infections. Dampness and Deficiency can also set in, triggering intestinal problems, abdominal swelling, and fluid retention.

These serious disturbances in the functioning of the body's Organ Systems occur in all forms of hepatitis, whether viral or triggered by drugs or environmental pollutants.

Additional Diagnoses Associated with Acute Hepatitis C

The following syndromes may appear in association with acute hepatitis and persist in chronic hepatitis as well:

Liver/Gallbladder Damp Heat

Relevant symptoms to HCV: bright yellow face/eyes, fever, costal pain (pain along rib cage), jaundice, nausea
Pulse: wiry and/or slippery
Tongue: red with greasy yellow coating

Spleen Damp Heat

Relevant symptoms to HCV: bright yellow face, abdominal pain, nausea, jaundice, fever, decreased appetite
Pulse: slippery/fast
Tongue: red with yellow greasy coating

Spleen Damp Cold

Relevant symptoms to HCV: sallow yellow face, abdominal pain, nausea, feels cold despite having a fever, decreased appetite
Pulse: slippery/tight
Tongue: pale with greasy white coating

DIAGNOSES ASSOCIATED WITH CHRONIC HEPATITIS C

Syndromes and symptoms may include those associated with acute hepatitis and the following syndromes as well.

Excess syndromes associated with chronic hepatitis C are as follows:

Liver Qi Stagnation

Symptoms relevant to HCV: fatigue, pain in the area of the rib cage, fullness in the abdomen, nausea, flatulence/bloating, increased liver enzymes, swollen liver and spleen
Pulse: wiry
Tongue: purplish or normal with thin white coat

Deficiency syndromes associated with chronic hepatitis C are as follows:

Spleen Qi Deficiency

Symptoms relevant to HCV: fatigue, abdominal tenderness, nausea/queasiness, lack of appetite, muscle weakness, loose stools
Pulse: deficient
Tongue: pale, swollen with toothmarks

Liver Yin Deficiency

Symptoms relevant to HCV: dryness of eyes, nails, throat, and mouth; fatigue; blurry vision; dizziness; muscle spasms; reddish cheeks and eyes; numb limbs; quick temper
Pulse: thin, deficient, wiry, rapid
Tongue: reddish sides

Qi Deficiency (General)

Symptoms relevant to HCV: fatigue, bleeding (such as purpura), leg edema, ascites
Pulse: deficient
Tongue: pale, swollen

Yin Deficiency (General)

Symptoms relevant to HCV: fatigue, reddish cheeks, night sweats, afternoon fevers or hot flashes, restlessness, night wakefulness
Pulse: thin, deficient, rapid
Tongue: reddish or with a red tip

The following Deficiency syndrome is often associated with cirrhosis:

Xue (Blood) Deficiency

Symptoms relevant to cirrhosis: pale and lusterless face, general dryness, normalized enzymes, shrunken liver
Pulse: deficient and thready/hollow if loss of blood
Tongue: pale

The following Excess syndrome is often associated with liver cancer (in addition to deficiency syndromes):

Xue (Blood) Stagnation

Symptoms relevant to liver cancer: sharp stabbing pain along the side of the torso, abdomen hurts with movement
Pulse: choppy or wiry (with pain)
Tongue: purple or purple sides

Another Path to Diagnosis of Hepatitis

In Chinese medicine one of the traditions of diagnostic science for epidemic diseases is based on the concept of the four levels of Warm Disease. These levels are identified as the superficial, outer level known as Wei or Protective Qi, Qi, Jing, and Xue.

In hepatitis, pathogenic Heat—either Toxic Heat or Damp Heat—enters the body on the level of Wei Qi. It may then penetrate to the levels of Qi, Jing, and Xue. It can inhabit more than one level at once and may manifest different syndromes and symptoms within each level. In this way, Heat may begin at the surface of the body and may penetrate to deeper levels, ultimately creating severe and end-stage disease.

Furthermore, it is also the case that all of the various Chinese medicine diagnoses mentioned previously in this book can manifest at one or more of the four levels of Warm Disease. Therefore, the herbal formulas that are used for treating hepatitis through the diagnostic process of Warm Disease are very similar to those used for diagnoses previously discussed in this chapter. For more detailed explanations refer to traditional Chinese medicine texts.

Home HCV Test

In the spring of 1999, the Food and Drug Administration approved an at-home HCV test called the Home Access Hepatitis C Check Test Service. It helps people determine if they have been exposed to the virus and offers them counseling and referral to appropriate medical care. The blood test is sent to a lab, and four to five days after receiving the sample, the lab reports the results.

The federal government has initiated the Hepatitis C Lookback Program, through which hundreds of thousands of people receive letters from blood banks and hospitals informing them that they may have been exposed to hepatitis C during blood transfusions prior to 1992. For people without access to free tests or a test covered by insurance, the $69.95 HCV test may offer them an easy way to determine if they have been infected with HCV. Over the next few years more companies are expected to offer this service, but for now only Home Access is FDA approved. For information on the test call 1-888-888-HEPC or check out the Web site at www.homeaccess.com.

6

Complications and Coinfections

THROUGH THE LONG, slow, often hidden life of the hepatitis C virus, the constant—if unremarkable—inflammation of the liver can create some serious complications.

Accumulated scar tissue in the liver can keep the organ from fulfilling its duties as head nutritionist and eventually prevent it from manufacturing or assembling vital building blocks, such as proteins, that are essential for the body's overall health. This same scarring can eventually block important veins and arteries, damaging the kidneys and even the brain. At the same time, for reasons not altogether clear, chronic liver disease can wreak havoc on the immune system, leading to an increased risk of various infections and making the body more prone to autoimmune diseases in which the body attacks its own healthy cells. The autoimmune complications that develop are most likely to affect the skin, thyroid gland, kidney, blood vessels, and joints. The wise management of chronic hepatitis C is designed to avoid development of complications.

Coinfection is also a problem for those who have chronic hepatitis C. Forty percent of those who are HIV positive also have HCV. One to 3 percent of those coinfected with HIV and HCV subsequently contract hepatitis B, with devastating consequences.

The smartest approach to avoiding coinfection is to get vaccinated for hepatitis A and B as soon as you are diagnosed with either hepatitis C or HIV. You should also act to reduce your risk factors for the various infections by practicing safe sex. And if you cannot stop using IV drugs, you should adopt scrupulously clean injection habits. Do not reuse needles.

HCV SIDE EFFECTS AND COMPLICATIONS

Primary Side Effects

Fuzzy Thinking

Definition and Symptoms: Severe viral infections can often make it difficult to think clearly even if there are few other symptoms. In hepatitis C the initial viral onslaught can disturb thinking processes. Later, when other complications arise, the inability of the liver to clear toxins from the blood is associated with memory disturbances and other problems with mental functioning.

Associated Chinese Medicine Syndromes: Mental disturbances and confusion are often diagnosed as Shen disharmonies, Kidney Deficiency, and/or Heart Deficiency.

Depression

Definition and Symptoms: Depression is a common complication of chronic disease for both biochemical and emotional reasons. Biochemically, a long-term viral disease can cause changes in brain and hormone chemistry that trigger depression. Emotionally, the anxiety and stress a person feels about having a serious chronic illness can in itself lead to depression.

Associated Chinese Medicine Syndromes: Depression is associated with Liver Qi Stagnation or Heart Xue Deficiency leading to Shen disturbances and liver disorders.

Fibrosis

Definition and Symptoms: The hepatitis C virus attacks the liver's cells and causes inflammation. This persistent irritation of the tissue can cause scarring. Scar tissue that replaces healthy liver tissue is called fibrosis.

Associated Chinese Medicine Syndromes: Fibrosis and its symptoms are associated with Qi Stagnation leading to Xue Stagnation. When fibrosis and cirrhosis reduce the size of the liver, then Xue Deficiency has set in.

Progressive Complications of Fibrosis

Cirrhosis

Definition and Symptoms: Cirrhosis is caused by the destruction of liver cell integrity and extensive fibrosis. In the early stages of cirrhosis, the liver is not yet damaged by compound complications; this early stage is called compensated cirrhosis. People with this level of cirrhosis have a survival rate of 91 percent at five years, but the rate falls to 79 percent at ten years as the liver disease progresses. For those who develop complications from cirrhosis such as liver failure or portal hypertension (called decompensated cirrhosis), the five-year survival rate is less than 50 percent. Liver failure from cirrhosis is a serious risk for these people.

These are the warning signs of liver failure:

- swollen feet
- muscle loss
- swollen abdomen (ascites)
- confusion
- progressive memory loss
- difficulty sleeping during the night and increased sleeping during the day
- vomiting blood
- passing blood
- purple or black bowel movements
- yellow eyes and/or skin
- "thin" blood caused by clotting disorders
- low albumin—less than 3.5 mg/dL
- high bilirubin—more than 2 mg/dL
- low platelets—less than 100,000
- low cholesterol—less than 100 mg/dL
- flapping of the extended hands (asterixis)

Progressive Complications of Cirrhosis

High Bilirubin Levels

Definition and Symptoms: Bilirubin is a waste product—actually an organic salt—that comes from the breakdown of heme, the main oxygen-transporting molecule in red blood cells. If liver damage prevents it from being converted into a water-soluble substance, this yellowish liquid acts as a toxin and produces jaundice.

Associated Chinese Medicine Syndromes: The symptoms associated with high bilirubin levels indicate Damp Heat in the Liver, and Spleen Organ Systems and Cold Damp in the Spleen Organ System.

Low Glucose Levels

Definition and Symptoms: The liver balances the body's blood levels of sugars, such as glucose, and provides a continuous supply of these sugars to the brain, muscles, and other tissues. If the liver is functioning below par and there is not a sufficient or regular supply of essential sugars, then muscle wasting and brain malfunction can occur.

Associated Chinese Medicine Syndromes: If low glucose levels cause fatigue and you feel better after eating small amounts and often feel worse after eating big, heavy meals, the diagnosis is probably Spleen Deficiency. Dizziness and light-headedness are symptoms of Qi and Xue Deficiencies.

Low Albumin Levels

Definition and Symptoms: Albumin, a blood protein manufactured in the liver, is essential to maintain a healthy circulation. Low levels allow fluid to leak out of the blood vessels, causing swelling of the legs and abdomen.

Associated Chinese Medicine Syndromes: Disturbances in water metabolism that lead to swelling are associated with Triple Burner disharmonies and Kidney and Spleen Deficiencies.

High Ammonia Levels

Definition and Symptoms: Ammonia is a by-product of protein metabolism, and high blood levels indicate the liver is not cleaning dangerous toxins from the blood. High levels can cause mental confusion and may lead to another serious complication: encephalopathy, a state of mental confusion or drowsiness.

Associated Chinese Medicine Syndromes: The kind of mental confusion associated with high ammonia levels is an indication of Shen disharmony, and since aspects of the Shen are housed in the Liver Organ System, it also indicates the presence of serious Liver Organ System disease syndromes.

Lowered Cholesterol Levels

Definition and Symptoms: The liver is the main source of serum cholesterol, which is essential for the production of hormones and for a healthy cardiovascular system. A cholesterol level that is too low is a sign of liver malfunction and indicates a general decline in health. Low levels also make the body more vulnerable to the potential toxicity of certain medications.

Associated Chinese Medicine Syndromes: Low cholesterol leading to diminished sexual desire is associated with Kidney Disharmony.

Abnormal INR or Prothrombin Time: Changes in Blood Clotting

Definition and Symptoms: The liver is the organ responsible for producing proteins that control blood clotting. When scarring in the liver damages the cells that produce clotting factors, INR levels and prothrombin time—the time needed for blood to coagulate—increase. As a result, bleeding is difficult to stop and small blood vessels may leak blood into the esophagus, stomach, and bowel, particularly when the skin is irritated or bruised or as a result of surgery.

Associated Chinese Medicine Syndromes: Bleeding problems that show up as spots on the skin are caused by the Spleen Not Holding the Xue Within the Vessels. Bloody stools are a sign of severe Spleen Deficiency with Sinking Qi.

Portal Hypertension

Definition and Symptoms: Cirrhosis-related scar tissue constricts the sinusoids, the tiny veins that branch off from the portal vein and run throughout the liver. Slowly, as the blood flow through them is cut off, blood backs up in the larger portal vein, increasing pressure until hypertension develops. This sets off a cascade of trauma to other vessels, which become dilated by the force of the blood backing up and increasing pressure—most commonly in the spleen, esophagus, and stomach. This results in the accumulation of fluid in the abdomen (ascites) and may cause veins in the esophagus, and stomach to rupture, causing severe bleeding. Portal hypertension eventually develops in those with progressive cirrhosis.

Complications of Portal Hypertension

Ascites

Definition and Symptoms: Portal hypertension and low albumin levels cause this serious complication. It triggers fluid retention in the abdominal cavity (often very large amounts).

Associated Chinese Medicine Syndromes: Ascites is associated with severe Spleen Qi and Yang Deficiency and Triple Burner disharmonies.

Spontaneous Bacterial Peritonitis

Definition and Symptoms: This condition occurs when the ascites fluid becomes infected, and it can lead to rapid liver failure.

Associated Chinese Medicine Syndromes: Such intense infections, when accompanied by fever, are a result of Toxic and Damp Heat invading various Organ Systems and Essential Substances.

Gastrointestinal Bleeding, Vomiting, or Passing Blood

Definition and Symptoms: Bleeding from the veins and capillaries in the stomach and esophagus is a life-threatening condition. It is often triggered by portal hypertension, which puts pressure on the vessels, making them rupture. The surgery required to stop the bleeding is delicate and risky, and the bleeding is difficult to stop. There is also an increased risk of duodenal and stomach ulcers in people with cirrhosis.

Associated Chinese Medicine Syndromes: The diagnosis for these types of complications is Spleen Qi Deficiency leading to the Spleen Not Holding the Xue Within the Vessels. As the condition becomes more and more severe, it becomes a sign of Xue Stagnation.

Digestive Problems, Hemorrhoids, and Leg Swelling

Definition and Symptoms: As the portal vein is blocked, digestion slows down and there is a decrease in the delivery of bile to the gut. As a result, fat digestion becomes more and more difficult. Deficiencies in vitamins A, D, and K develop. (They are fat-soluble vitamins. Vitamin E, which is also fat soluble, is not as much of a problem because so much is available in our diet.) Obstructed blood flow can also trigger hemorrhoids and cause fluid accumulation in the legs.

Associated Chinese Medicine Syndromes: These complications are associated with severe Spleen and Stomach Deficiencies. When gas and pain are also a factor, Qi Stagnation is the likely diagnosis. If swelling affects the abdomen (as in ascites) or the whole body, then Spleen Qi Deficiency and Triple Burner disharmony are the usual diagnoses.

Hormone Imbalances

Definition and Symptoms: Cirrhosis and portal hypertension alter gonadal hormone synthesis in the liver and can cause elevated estrogen levels. In men, elevated estrogen levels can trigger spider veins, testicular atrophy, development of breasts, loss of body hair, lower libido, and sexual dysfunction.

Associated Chinese Medicine Syndromes: Spider veins are associated with the Spleen Not Holding the Xue Within the Vessels. When the veins appear on the face, that is also associated with a Yin Deficiency. Testicular atrophy is a Kidney Jing Deficiency; the formation of breasts is a Liver Qi Stagnation problem; loss of body hair is associated with Xue and Kidney Deficiencies. In women, elevated estrogen levels may increase PMS symptoms associated with Liver Qi Stagnation. They may also cause a lack of sexual desire, associated with Kidney Deficiency, or painful periods, which are associated with Qi and Xue Stagnation, or Qi and Xue Deficiencies. Irregular periods may be associated with Kidney, Spleen, Heart, and Xue Deficiencies.

Encephalopathy

Definition and Symptoms: Encephalopathy is a condition caused by naturally occurring chemical toxins that remain circulating in the bloodstream because the HCV-damaged liver cannot properly clear them out. These toxins trigger neurological and brain changes, which in turn cause memory lapses, confused thinking, sleep disturbances, and, in extreme cases, coma. There are many toxins involved, but the one most commonly measured is ammonia. Zinc levels are also frequently measured to determine if there is a deficiency, which may worsen the symptoms of encephalopathy. Zinc deficiencies are common in liver disease, and zinc is required to clear ammonia from the blood.

Associated Chinese Medicine Syndromes: Mental confusion and memory lapses are associated with Heart Xue Deficiency, Heart Fire, and Spleen and Kidney Deficiency. Waking up in the night is often a result of Yin Deficiency, and severe Qi and Yang Deficiency is the diagnosis when coma occurs.

Pruritis

Definition and Symptoms: Pruritis is a condition characterized by chronic skin itchiness. It happens when the liver cannot remove toxins from the blood (and, consequently, the skin). Since antihistamines and lotions have no effect on hepatitis-related pruritis, an incapacitating bout can be reason enough for a liver transplant.

Associated Chinese Medicine Syndromes Pruritis is the direct result of Toxic Heat as it moves more deeply into the body.

Muscle Wasting Due to Low Blood Sugar and Malnutrition

Definition and Symptoms: Severe cirrhosis can lead to muscle wasting, which causes weakness, fatigue, and inactivity. The best remedy is a moderate amount of weight-bearing exercises combined with a healthy diet plan of five meals per day of complex carbohydrates and doctor-recommended supplements. Unfortunately, growth hormone, which can help rebuild muscle mass, is toxic to the infected liver.

Associated Chinese Medicine Syndromes: Severe Spleen Deficiency is associated with loss of muscle mass and weakness.

Liver Cancer (HCC)

Definition and Symptoms: Liver cancer, also called hepatocellular carcinoma or HCC, is the ninth most common form of cancer in this country: Approximately six thousand cases are diagnosed in the United States each year. The disease is more common in men than in women.

People who develop cirrhosis have a 20 percent chance of also developing HCC over a period of ten years. When someone infected with HCV drinks alcohol, the risk of developing liver cancer doubles. If cirrhosis is present, it becomes an even more dangerous assault on the liver.

In other parts of the world, such as Africa, Southeast Asia, and China, HCC is a major health problem, making up to 75 percent of the cancer cases seen in those areas. This difference is thought to be due to the much higher percentage of carriers of hepatitis B virus (from 10 to 20 percent of the population in those regions), compared to 0.5 percent in Caucasians in the United States. Being a carrier of hepatitis B antigens (even after the acute attack is passed) increases the risk of developing HCC by 200 percent!

Primary liver cancer is hard to detect at the beginning. The first symptom is usually pain that goes from the abdomen to the back and shoulder. Weight loss is common. Sometimes patients have episodes of severe pain, fever, and nausea. Rapidly deteriorating health, weakness, fever, tenderness, and jaundice may lead doctors to suspect liver cancer.

If you have cirrhosis, it is a good idea to have a blood test for cancer (AFP—alpha-fetoprotein) and an ultrasound of the liver every six months. If liver cancer is caught early, liver transplantation can be a very effective cure.

Associated Chinese Medicine Syndromes: Liver cancer is associated with Qi and Xue Deficiency, which may lead to severe Xue Stagnation.

Immune Complexes and Autoimmune Diseases Associated with HCV

Definition and Symptoms: Autoimmune diseases occur when the body's disease defense system (the immune system) mistakenly identifies healthy cells in the body as sources of potential disease. The immune cells then attack and kill the healthy cells in a misguided attempt to protect the body from an imagined disease. The result is a hard-to-stop onslaught that wreaks havoc in a wide range of systems and in various parts of the body.

The hepatitis C virus may induce an autoimmune liver disease and HCV infection appears to be associated with autoimmune thyroiditis, lichen planus, salivary gland inflammation, and possibly other forms of autoimmune disease.

Lichen Planus

Definition and Symptoms: This autoimmune skin disorder is associated with general liver dysfunction. It is characterized by clusters of irregular bumps with flat tops and generally appears on the wrists, shins, lower back, and genital areas. The condition is not painful but may cause itching. The itching can be treated with topical creams.

Associated Chinese Medicine Syndromes: Heat in the Xue and Damp Heat.

Raynaud's Syndrome

Definition and Symptoms: A painful condition that can turn the nose, ears, hands, and feet a cold blue and, sometimes, white. It may result in severe skin damage and ulcers.

Associated Chinese Medicine Syndromes: This syndrome is associated with either Liver Qi Stagnation, in which the energy of the body stays in the interior and doesn't move to the extremities, or Yang Deficiency, in which the person is thoroughly cold but particularly in the extremities.

Thyroiditis

Definition and Symptoms: Data suggest that infection with HCV increases the risk of thyroid inflammation, which can result in hyper- or hypothyroidism (elevated or lowered production of the thyroid hormone). Taking interferon may worsen this vulnerability to thyroid disorders, although the drug may also be the main cause. If thyroiditis is drug-induced and caught early, the thyroid will return to normal once interferon is stopped. If interferon therapy is continued, thyroid medication is needed. Symptoms of thyroid deficiency include fatigue, depression, constipation, weight gain, poor memory, coldness, and dry skin.

Associated Chinese Medicine Syndromes: Coldness is a Qi Yang Deficiency; itching is the result of Heat in Xue or a Xue Deficiency leading to Heat in Xue. Poor memory is sometimes related to Shen disturbances. Depression is related to Shen disturbances and Liver Qi Stagnation. Fatigue can be related to Qi Deficiency or Stagnation, Dampness, or Xue Deficiency.

Immune Complexes Associated with HCV

Definition and Symptoms: Immune complexes are giant molecules that form when pieces of the HCV virus clump together with immune system antibodies. These floating barges of immune system-related material—called cryoglobulins—travel through the circulatory system. When they enter small passageways in the kidneys, the joints, or the brain, they get stuck, causing inflammation and pain and disrupting organ functions.

Cryoglobulins can be found in up to 40 percent of people infected with HCV and may explain the muscle and joint aches and pains that are so common in hepatitis C. A small percentage of people (around 2 percent) actually develop tissue damage that can be found on physical examination or laboratory analysis. This damage includes a red or purple raised rash (leukocytoclastic vascullitis, or palpable purpura), and may result in damage to the skin, kidney, eyes, nerves, brain, and heart. These oversized molecules may also cause intestinal disturbances, sinus stuffiness, and fuzzy thinking. Some people report painful feelings in their extremities, and the condition has been associated with a neuropathy, a nerve disease that triggers pain or numbness.

Why the immune system goes awry when HCV appears on the scene is unknown. The newest research suggests that it may occur only in people with a genetic predisposition which makes them vulnerable to the negative impact of HCV on the immune system. Some researchers suspect that the HCV virus triggers immune dysfunction, not unlike the assault on the immune system associated with HIV.

Cryoglobulinemia

Definition and Symptoms: Cryoglobulinemia is the name for the disorder caused by oversized protein molecules called cryoglobulins. This disorder triggers no symptoms at all for almost 80 percent of those who develop it; the other 20 percent experience fatigue, joint pain, and a red rash, usually appearing on the feet and shins. People with cryoglobulinemia are considered at higher risk for the development of B-cell lymphomas.

The standard treatment for cryoglobulinemia is interferon therapy. In severe cases it may also be necessary to undergo plasmapheresis, a filtering process that removes the offending chunks of viral protein from the blood.

Associated Chinese Medicine Syndromes: Immune dysfunction and resulting symptoms are often a reflection of Qi Deficiency, Xue Deficiency, the Spleen

Not Holding the Xue Within the Vessels, Bi Syndrome (painful joints), and Xue and Damp Stagnation.

Complications of Cryoglobulinemia

B-cell Non-Hodgkin's Lymphoma

Definition and Symptoms: After a prolonged period of cryoglobulinemia, this special type of lymph node tumor may develop.

Associated Chinese Medicine Syndromes: If the tumor is in the brain, it may be associated with a Shen disturbance. If the nodules are hard, it is Xue Stagnation. If they are soft, it is Qi Stagnation or Phlegm Stagnation.

Glomerulonephritis

Definition and Symptoms: When the clumped-together molecules block the vessels in the kidney, inflammation, or glomerulonephritis, results. This can cause kidney insufficiency, protein loss from the kidney, and, eventually, kidney failure and dialysis. A kidney transplant may become necessary.

Because of these possible risks, everyone with hepatitis C should undergo a blood test for creatinine, which is an indicator of kidney function. It is also a good idea to have a urinalysis to see if protein is leaking into the urine.

Associated Chinese Medicine Syndromes: Dry mouth and lack of tears are associated with Dryness syndromes; when there is fluid accumulation and kidney failure, the fluid metabolism cycle that is controlled by the Triple Burner, Kidney, Lung, and Spleen Systems is disturbed.

Leukocytoclastic Vasculitis (Purpura) and Leg Ulcers

Definition and Symptoms: An accumulation of immune complexes in the small capillaries in the legs or other skin areas may cause circulation problems that result in a raised purple rash. Leg ulcers may also occur from ruptured vessels in the thighs, calves, or around the ankles. These problems may be confused with the signs of kidney dysfunction; anytime a red or purple rash appears on the lower extremities, it is important that a kidney assessment be made.

Associated Chinese Medicine Syndromes: Ruptured blood vessels and skin symptoms are triggered by the Spleen Not Holding the Xue Within the Vessels and Xue Stagnation or Heat in the Xue.

Cerebral Vasculitis and Associated Neuropathy

Definition and Symptoms: Inflammation of the blood vessels in the brain caused by oversize immune complex molecules circulating in the bloodstream. This can cause neuropathy, or nerve damage, which may become irreversible.

Associated Chinese Medicine Syndromes: When the brain function is affected, the basic diagnosis is usually a Shen disturbance. When depression is present, it is Qi Stagnation. When there is severe sharp pain, Xue Stagnation is also involved.

Fibromyalgia

Definition and Symptoms: This term describes a syndrome of aches, pains, and stiffness between joints and the fibrous connective tissues (ligaments).

Associated Chinese Medicine Syndromes: Qi Stagnation, Damp Stagnation with underlying Spleen Deficiency, and Bi syndrome (joint pain) are the associated syndromes.

Arthralgias

Definition and Symptoms: Although arthritis is a rare complication of HCV, arthralgias such as joint and muscle aches and pains, possibly caused by the immune complex molecules, are common.

Associated Chinese Medicine Syndromes: Such symptoms are associated with what is known as the Bi syndrome; they may also be caused by Wind Damp, Wind Heat, or Wind Cold invading the joints.

Diabetes

Definition and Symptoms: Diabetes may result from an HCV-triggered autoimmune dysfunction, which destroys the cells in the pancreas that produce insulin. It can also result from liver damage that blocks the body's ability to regulate sugars (particularly glycogen) and insulin.

Associated Chinese Medicine Syndromes: Chinese dietary therapy is the first step in regulating blood sugar levels. Other treatments depend on the symptoms that are present. Increased hunger but no interest in eating is probably a sign of a Spleen Yin Deficiency. Several Kidney and Spleen Deficiencies are related to fatigue, mood swings, and thirst.

HCV COINFECTIONS

Many people with HCV are at risk for or already have HIV. In fact, 40 percent of those who have been diagnosed with HIV also have HCV, and there is every reason to fear that the percentage will increase over the next decade. In addition, people with HCV are at additional risk for other forms of hepatitis, particularly hepatitis B and D. These coinfections create serious medical crises and raise many complicated treatment issues that often leave the person with the coinfection feeling torn between two unsatisfactory treatment options: Do nothing or treat one of the viruses and risk worsening the other. That is why anyone infected with HIV or HCV should be vaccinated against hepatitis A and B, and why anyone with HIV should be tested for HCV and HBV. Early detection offers the best advantage in treating any coinfection.

HCV and HIV

Twenty percent of people with HIV who contract HCV cannot develop antibodies to HCV because HIV has devastated their immune systems. This means that the body is unable to mount any fight at all against hepatitis. And even for the 80 percent of HIV-infected people who do produce antibodies when exposed to HCV, the combination of HIV and HCV doubles the risk that they will sustain severe liver damage from the hepatitis infection. Another possible hazard: If a coinfected person is taking combination therapy of protease inhibitors and other antivirals to treat the HIV, the HCV-infected liver may not be able to detoxify the medication, and the side effects from it—including liver damage—may be increased.

Making the decision about which virus to treat first is also difficult. In people with both HCV and HIV infections, the benefits of therapy for hepatitis C have not been clearly proved, and the repercussions of combining medications for both diseases must be taken into consideration.

For the individual faced with this dilemma, choices are difficult and can be made only with early detection and consultation with all involved physicians. The latest information can be found on the Internet at www.HIVandHepatitis.com, as well as in articles written by Misha Cohen found at www.hepcchallenge.org.

HCV and HAV/HBV

Coinfection with another form of hepatitis places an enormous strain on the liver and speeds the development of serious liver disease and associated complications. The most common coinfection is between HCV and HBV. Almost 2 percent of those with HCV also have an active case of HBV and almost 60 percent have had HBV at some time in the past and are now immune. It is quite difficult to treat coinfected patients, partly because there is precious little data to support the diagnosis and treatment for these groups, and because there are no therapies for treating acute hepatitis A or B, except for rest, fluids, and patience. The best possible approach is probably to treat the "dominant" infection, as determined by blood tests.

Chinese Medicine Notes

In Chinese medicine both HIV and HCV are associated with Toxic Heat, and their related syndromes and symptoms can be treated simultaneously. There is no danger from conflicting therapies. The practitioner will arrive at a diagnosis that embraces the whole body's response to the dual infection, and therapy is tailored to respond to whatever complex syndromes the two infections produce in the mind/body/spirit. For detailed information on using Chinese medicine in conjunction with Western therapies to treat HIV and its related condition, see Dr. Cohen's book, *The HIV Wellness Source Book.*

TREATMENT CHOICES

WESTERN MEDICAL TREATMENT OPTIONS FROM
ROBERT G. GISH, M.D.

Hepatitis C is a daily challenge to those who are infected with HCV—and to those who are concerned with finding treatments and cures that will improve quality of life and clear the virus from the body. Every morning when I wake up I am hit with the enormity of work there is to be done to eliminate this disease.

Part of that challenge is to educate people about the risks of hepatitis C. I believe there are a huge number of people with hepatitis C who are undiagnosed (probably close to 5 million). The health-care community must help people recognize if they are potential carriers and need to be screened for the virus. This is the best way to see that those who are infected and need treatment are treated as soon as possible to prevent the unintentional spread of the virus to others.

Another aspect of the challenge is finding the best treatment solutions. Presently, the drug treatment that we can provide is not as good as we might wish. Many people have a type of hepatitis C that is resistant to interferon and ribavirin, the mainstay of treatment; and ribavirin, an antiviral that is used in combination with interferon, is rarely effective when taken by itself. They both produce serious side effects. And for about one-half of people infected, they do not clear the virus.

That's why it is particularly important to address quality of life issues for people with hepatitis C. Problems such as a decline in social and sexual functioning, interruption of the sleep cycle, mental fuzziness, and general aches and pains can make every day a difficult challenge. We have medications that can ease some of these problems, but the lack of an effective cure for many people means that health-care providers and patients alike are looking for additional ways to manage hepatitis C. They want to change how the virus affects their life. That is where Chinese medicine makes a major contribution. Although herbs do not cure hepatitis C, they may modulate the inflammatory response that damages the liver and, more important, improve the quality of life for those patients infected with HCV, or improve the outcomes of treatment. Herbs are also useful in the management of pain, digestive problems, general problems with mental clarity, and depression. And various other Chinese medicine practices may help people improve their sense of well-being.

As Western medicine pursues the ultimate cure, treatment must push forward to make the everyday life of each person with hepatitis C as rewarding as possible. In this effort I am guided by one simple belief: Life is short enough as it is, it should also be good.

7

Western Drug Therapy for Hepatitis C

Your doctor's told you, "You have hepatitis C."

So now what?

Prompt evaluation and treatment, that's what. And, given certain restrictions, the sooner the better.

For people who have not yet developed symptoms of liver failure and have moderate, progressive liver disease, treatment options include a combination of interferon and ribavirin, and/or Chinese medicine. This provides the best shot for improving quality of life, clearing the virus from the bloodstream, and halting the progression of the disease.

Despite the frequent ineffectiveness and sometimes serious side effects of Western medications, treatment with them does clear the virus from the blood and the liver (a cure) for a meaningful percentage of people—up to 46 percent of those on combination therapy. Patients with genotype 2 and 3 may have cure rates as high as 70 to 90 percent while genotype 1 patients typically have a sustained response in only 40 to 42 percent of patients. African Americans and patients who are immune-suppressed have an even worse chance of cure.

Many Western doctors feel the potential benefits of interferon and ribavirin outweigh the risks and disadvantages, because 20 to 30 percent of all those with hepatitis C will develop cirrhosis—which is truly debilitating and potentially life-threatening. In fact, hepatitis C–induced, end-stage liver disease is the most common reason for liver transplants in the United States. Individuals infected with HCV who develop cirrhosis have a much higher risk of also going on to developing liver cancer.

CURRENT TREATMENT OPTIONS

Interferon

Interferon is a protein that is produced and secreted by special immune cells and acts as an antiviral, immune-regulating chemical. When it enters the bloodstream and attaches to infected cells, it interferes with the hepatitis C virus's ability to replicate. In addition, interferon appears to shore up the immune system's disease-fighting T helper cells so that they are strong enough to kill off the hepatitis C viruses.

When used as medication, interferon is either genetically engineered or a synthetic replica of the body's protein. Originally licensed in 1986 to treat hairy cell leukemia, the FDA okayed its use in treating hepatitis C in 1991. The five interferons are presently approved in the United States are: **interferon alfa-2b** (Intron® A) and **PEG-Intron®** (pegylated interferon alfa-2b), Schering-Plough, Kenilworth, New Jersey; **interferon alfa-2a** (Roferon-A®), **PEGASYS®** (pegylated interferon alfa-2a), Hoffman La Roche Laboratories, Basle, Switzerland and **consensus interferon,** also called interferon alfacon—(**Infergen**) from Valeant Pharmaceuticals International. These long-acting, time-release forms of interferon, called pegylated (PEG) interferon, keep interferon blood levels high for three to ten days, delivering a more sustained punch. Injections are only needed once per week.

Today, using these various products, treatment has evolved to include higher dose interferon therapy, daily therapy, time-released doses, and with the current standard, combination of pegylated interferon and ribavirin. On the horizon, there are many other potentially useful treatments being developed.

When monotherapy with alpha interferon does work, it is usually in people who do not have fibrosis or cirrhosis, are infected with a genotype of HCV other than 1a or 1b, have viral loads of less than 2 million/ml, and have been infected with HCV for a relatively short period of time. Still, monotherapy remains the only option for those who cannot tolerate ribavirin (the antiviral medication used with interferon in combination therapy), and alternate forms of interferon may be used as monotherapy if combination therapy has been tried and was ineffective.

Why can't interferon do a better job of clearing the virus from the body, when by all rights it should work? One theory, reported in *Archive of Virology*,[1] suggested that undiagnosed coinfection with chronic hepatitis B may be the reason that interferon treatment does not work in some cases. They suggest that even if the interferon does work against HCV, HBV remains active and continues to replicate, causing persistent symptoms of liver disease. Certain ethnic groups, such as African Americans, have a response rate that is much lower than other ethnic groups, which may be due to genetic defects in their immune system. Other reasons for nonresponse include increasing weight, noncompliance and nonadherance, alcohol use, immunosuppression with HIV or medications, fatty liver, and older age. High iron levels—a result of liver dysfunction—may also interfere with the effectiveness of interferon. Iron reduction therapy (phlebotomy or chelation) in combination with interferon has been studied, but the results have thus far been inconclusive.

Side Effects of Interferon

Up to 20 to 60 percent of all people who start out on interferon drop out because of the unpleasant and sometimes serious side effects, causing 10 to 40 percent to reduce their dosage. This dropout rate is much lower in the experienced practitioner's office. The impact of side effects is reduced if interferon is taken at night before going to bed, and the severity of the flu-like symptoms can be reduced by pretreatment with acetaminophen. Many new treatment options are available to treat side effects.

NOTE FROM DR. GISH:

Although high doses of acetaminophen can be liver toxic, it is still the safest pain remedy available if taken in doses of equal to or less than 2 grams a day—that's four extra-strength Tylenol. Ibuprofen is also safe, if you have no kidney disease or ulcers.

Initial side effects of interferon include:

- persistent flu-like symptoms
- nausea
- loss of energy
- depression
- loss of appetite
- worsening diabetes
- worsening of lipid problems
- hair loss
- weight loss

Long-term side effects include:

- fatigue
- bone marrow suppression and anemia
- neuropsychiatric effects such as:
    apathy
    cognitive changes

    irritability

    depression

- thyroiditis

To learn more about the side effects of ribavirin and interferon you should read the package insert and review information available on the Internet at the pharmaceutical companies' Web sites.

Ribavirin

Ribavirin is an antiviral medication, called a nucleoside analogue, that blocks the virus's ability to replicate and alters the immune system cells that fight viruses, making them more effective. It is the drug treatment choice these days, when used in conjunction with pegylated alpha interferons. Around 95 percent of people receiving treatment now start out on the combination therapy.

Although ribavirin alone has almost no direct effect on HCV replication, when teamed with pegylated interferon it produces a sustained reduction in viral load to undetectable levels in 54 to 56 percent of people who take it. (These are folks who are being treated for the first time. They have not taken interferon at some earlier date, and had it fail.)

Among people who had taken interferon and saw positive results while on the drug, but relapsed once they stopped taking it, combination therapy is 46 percent effective in long-term eradication of detectable viral load and normalizing of liver enzyme levels. After liver transplantation, among those who have a recurrence of hepatitis C, combination therapy seems to provide sustained improvement 24 percent of the time. And the two-drug cocktail offers a 20 to 40 percent positive response rate to people for whom interferon monotherapy had provided no benefit whatsoever. Other versions of nucleoside analogues are in development and promise to be even more effective.

Side Effects of Ribavirin

According to the Hepatitis Support Project, "In addition to the side effects of interferon, ribavirin can cause severe anemia. This anemia can be counteracted by the use of erythropoietin, a natural protein that boost red cell counts in the blood. Ribavirin is contraindicated for anyone with significant cardiovascular disease or pregnant women due to the fact it is teratogenic (can cause birth defects)." Additional side effects include cough, rash, and mental changes and nausea. A pregnancy test should always be taken before starting therapy and effective contraceptive practices are essential. Men who are taking combination therapy should also avoid fathering a child, as the sperm can carry the drugs and could result in birth defects. (See also page 99 for information regarding Milk Thistle or Silymarin.)

ASSESSING TREATMENT SUCCESS

Pegylated interferon and ribavirin combination do effectively clear (cure) the hepatitis C virus from the bloodstream of some people while and after they are taking the medication. Unfortunately, once treatment is stopped, the virus can reemerge. So, what constitutes a remission or cure of HCV? According to guidelines established by the National Institutes of Health, a sustained response to therapy is defined by a biochemical normalization of serum ALT levels (ALT less than 30 IU/mL) and a virologic response of undetectable HCV RNA levels (that's zero viral load) when measured six months after treatment is stopped. (Liver biopsy performed before and after treatment also can help demonstrate reduced liver inflammation and a positive response to drug therapy.) For patients with no virus six months after stopping therapy, less than 3 percent have emergence of virus in the blood or liver in the next 5 to 10 years.

WHO SHOULD BE TREATED?

Anyone with antibodies to HCV, HCV RNA (that is, a measurable viral load detected by a molecular test such as PCR, bDNA, or TMA test), elevated serum AST and ALT (liver enzyme) levels (any level over 30 IU/mL), and evidence of chronic hepatitis with fibrosis on liver biopsy, and with no contraindications to therapy, should be offered therapy with the combination of pegylated alpha interferon and ribavirin. Patients with normal liver enzymes can also be treated, but a liver biopsy may be even more helpful in this group, since they have a lower chance of progressive liver disease. Patients may also be treated without a liver biopsy, yet the biopsy allows the practitioner to allocate resources based on urgency of treatment (near-term risk of liver failure, death, or cancer).

The National Institutes of Health Consensus Development Conference Panel suggests treatment is definitely appropriate for people whose lab tests indicate moderate to severe inflammation, fibrosis, and liver cell necrosis (detected by a biopsy). People who reveal less severe inflammation, minor or no fibrosis or cell necrosis should receive treatment based on individual evaluation.

In all cases, however, treatment should not be contingent on whether or not that person has overt symptoms, how they contracted hepatitis C, the genotype of HCV with which they are infected, or their viral load levels.

If a liver biopsy reveals cirrhosis, drug therapy is possible as long as there are no signs of liver decompensation, such as ascites, persistent jaundice, wasting, variceal hemorrhage, or hepatic encephalopathy. For those in the early stages of cirrhosis, preliminary evidence shows that the time it takes to progress to liver failure or to receiving a transplant increase—and the chance of liver cancer may decrease—as a result of clearing the virus from the blood. For patients with signs of liver failure, treatment decisions must be made with a liver specialist and preferably with a transplant center

Those who are HCV positive and are sixty or older should be given treatment on a case-by-case basis. The benefits of treatment for these people have not been as well documented and side effects appear to be worse in older patients.

Children also must be individually evaluated for treatment: researchers have shown very high cure rates in children, but since their liver disease progression is slower, treatment is not as imperative. The safety of ribavirin for children has not been established.

In people with both HCV and HIV infection, therapy for hepatitis C may conflict with anti-HIV drugs, and there are now definitive studies showing the benefit of pegylated interferon and ribavirin with cure rates in the 30 to 40 percent range.

When HCV has triggered significant extrahepatic complications, such as nerve damage, rash from cryoglobulinemia, and often kidney damage due to glomerulonephritis, therapy with pegylated alpha interferon and ribavirin may lead to remission of symptoms and a cure of both HCV and the cryoglobulin disease. However, relapse after stopping therapy is seen and maintenance therapy is needed in some patients.

Some patients desire treatment based on perceptions of infectivity or fear of being ostracized from society. HCV can also interfere with relationships, specifically by inhibiting relationship development and intimacies.

Genotypes, Viral Load, and Therapy

Tests that reveal the magnitude of HCV infection—molecular tests (PCR, bDNA, TMA), tests for viral load, and liver enzyme tests for ALT and AST levels—allow you and your doctor to evaluate the risks and benefits of drug therapy. Remember, liver enzymes are not liver function tests, and the viral level or enzymes do not determine the level of liver damage. The best tests to determine if your liver is functioning normally are: bilirubin, albumin, and INR. If you have a low viral load—less then 500,000 IU/mL—you have an improved chance of sustaining a positive response to combination therapy, regardless of the genotype of HCV with which you are infected. In addition, determining the genotype and your viral load helps the doctor decide how long you need to remain on interferon as well as being the most powerful predictor of interferon response or cure. Treatment for genotype 2 is now as short as twelve weeks, genotype 3 for twenty-four to forty-eight weeks, and genotype 1 up to eighteen months.

WHO SHOULD NOT BE TREATED?

Monotherapy and combination therapy are not options outside of controlled scientific studies for anyone who has:

- clinically decompensated cirrhosis because of hepatitis C, unless being managed at a specialty liver-failure program
- a kidney, liver, heart, or other solid-organ transplant unless being managed at a specialty liver program
- clinical severe uncontrolled depression, and has a history of suicide attempts or chronic mental disease, unless cleared by a psychiatrist and undergoing active treatment. Alpha interferon has multiple neuropsychiatric effects. Prolonged therapy can cause marked irritability, anxiety, personality changes, depression, and even suicide or acute psychosis. Rarely, these changes are permanent. Patients particularly susceptible to these side effects are those with preexisting serious psychiatric conditions and with neurological disease.

Interferon therapy is also associated with relapse of drug use in people with a previous history of drug abuse. Alpha interferon should not be given to a patient who has only recently stopped alcohol or substance abuse unless in a controlled setting, such as a rehabilitation program or methadone treatment clinic. Strict abstinence from alcohol is recommended for all patients with HCV as well as during therapy with interferon. Marijuana has recently been shown to cause accelerated fibrosis in patients with HCV infection.

Alpha interferon therapy can induce autoantibodies, and a six- to twelve-month course triggers an autoimmune condition in about 2 percent of patients, particularly if they have an underlying susceptibility to autoimmunity (high levels of antinuclear or antithyroid antibodies, for instance). Autoimmune diseases such as rheumatoid arthritis or psoriasis often become more severe during interferon therapy and close monitoring of thyroid function must take place every six months or with the onset of any unusual symptom complex.

Alpha interferon suppresses bone marrow production of key cells. Therefore, patients with bone marrow-related disorders, such as low platelet count (below 75,000 cells/ mm3) or neutropenia (< 1,000 cells/ mm3), must be given drug therapy cautiously and have cell counts monitored frequently. Growth factors can be used to increase bone marrow counts.

Neither ribavirin nor interferon should be given to women considering pregnancy, nor should a man father a child while taking the drugs. Birth defects are a serious risk.

Ribavirin is contraindicated if a person has severe anemia, kidney dysfunction or disease, coronary artery or cerebrovascular disease, or is unable to practice birth control.

Ribavirin causes red cell hemolysis (disease of the red blood cells) to some degree or another in almost everyone who takes it. Therefore, anyone with a preexisting hemolysis or anemia (hemoglobin below 11 grams or hematocrit below 33 percent) should not receive ribavirin unless closely monitored, and the patient has access to erythropoietin, a growth factor that stimulates the bone marrow to produce red blood cells.

People with significant coronary or cerebral vascular disease should not receive ribavirin unless very closely monitored, as the anemia caused by treatment can trigger serious constriction of the blood vessels. Fatal heart attacks and strokes have been reported during combination therapy with alpha interferon and ribavirin.

The kidneys are largely responsible for excretion of ribavirin. People with renal disease can develop more severe hemolysis (a breaking down of the red blood cells) that can be life-threatening. Anyone who has serum creatinine above 2.0 mg/dL should not be treated with ribavirin.

Combination therapy should therefore be used with caution. Patients should be fully informed of the potential side effects before starting therapy. New side effects are being reported yearly in the literature, and all patients and practitioners must counsel patients about these risks prior to starting therapy.

ALTERNATIVE PHARMACEUTICAL THERAPIES

It is difficult to find a universally effective treatment for HCV because the virus mutates so rapidly that it can slide around any immune defenses that are set up. It's also hard to come up with a therapy that can be taken orally. It must not be harmful to the liver and yet it must still retain its ability to wage war against the virus in the liver. Most researchers are looking for combination therapies that can accomplish the task. Here is a look at the newest drugs that may be used with interferon to effectively slow down the rate of viral replication and mutation:

Other Immune Modulators

Crude thymus extracts (Thymic Fractions 1402 A, Immunoplex 402, Thymosin fraction 5, Thymosin alpha-1) are cytokines—that is, immune system T cells that are produced by the thymus gland and battle against viral infections. They appear to restrain the progression of chronic hepatitis. Trials combining these agents with interferon are underway: Thymosin alpha-1 is an immune cell product that appears naturally in the bloodstream of people infected with the hepatitis viruses. Researchers are experimenting with using these immune cells along with interferon and ribavirin to fight hepatitis C. New forms of interferon, including those bound to albumin, may allow injections monthly to treat hepatitis C. Isatorabine, a new immunomodulator, is also in clinical trials.

Viral Blocks: Stopping Replication and Protein Production

There are three enzymes that are crucial to the hepatitis C virus's protein production and replication: proteinase (this is the same as protease), helicase, and RNA polymerase. An enormous amount of research is going into finding ways to keep them from doing their work. Without their help, the hepatitis C virus would be unable to multiply in the body and eventually it would die off.

RNA-Dependent HCV RNA Polymerase Inhibitors

Scientists are searching for some way to prevent the hepatitis C virus from reproducing. In addition, they would like to find a way to prevent HCV from mutating into a new form, which would also help the immune system clear the virus and prevent chronic infection. To accomplish these goals, researchers have turned their attention to the HCV RNA-dependent RNA polymerase—the enzyme that controls the replication of the virus's entire genetic makeup. If a drug can be designed that stops the polymerase enzyme from putting together the ever-mutating genetic puzzle, which creates a new viral strain, then the disease could be stopped. Idenix Pharmaceuticals (Cambridge, Massachusetts) has a new compound NM 283, a polymerase inhibitor that is showing promising early results. Other companies are working actively in this area.

Helicase Inhibitors

The HCV helicase enzyme is involved in the unwinding or unfolding of the HCV RNA structure when it moves toward mutation. Blocking this development is currently the aim of intense study and drug development.

Proteinase (Protease) Inhibitors

In the process of getting ready to reproduce itself, the HC virus makes long strips of protein. It is the protease enzyme's job to snip the strips into sections, each with its own specialized function. If the enzyme can be prevented from doing its tailoring job, the protein won't be divided into its working parts, and the virus will be left without the material it needs to synthesize more viruses. Vertex, Schering-Plough, and other companies have medications entering phase III studies with theses compounds in the near future.

Anti-sense Oligonucleotides

A no-nonsense approach to preventing amino acids from being assembled into viral proteins—oligonucleotides bind to the viral RNA, usurping the place of the amino acids, and preventing replication and mutation. The problem is that the oligonucleotide is a huge molecule and is hard for the body to absorb; scientists have yet to figure out how to get it into the bloodstream effectively.

ON THE HORIZON

Although this therapy does not have any great antiviral effect by itself, there has been some interesting preliminary research. According to a report in the *Journal of Interferon Research,* in interferon-unresponsive patients, the addition of 600 mg tid of oral NAC (N-acetyl cysteine) may help enhance the effectiveness of interferon. NAC, a glutathione precursor, resulted in a steady decrease of ALT values in all patients, with complete normalization in 41 percent of cases after five to six months of combined therapy. The authors conclude that NAC enhanced the response to interferon in chronic hepatitis C, and suggest that further studies were needed to determine whether antioxidant therapy would be useful in conjunction with interferon treatment of hepatitis C.[2]

BEYOND DRUG TREATMENT

If drug treatment fails to stop the progression of liver disease, or if hepatitis C is diagnosed too late in the lifeline of the disease to make drug therapy possible, then liver transplant offers the best hope for management of the disease and recovery from cirrhosis and associated complications.

A liver transplant is not a cure, however. Hepatitis C infects the new transplanted liver 100 percent of the time and there is a 25 percent risk of developing cirrhosis within five years (much higher than in native livers), because the immunosuppressive drugs you have to take to prevent rejection of an implanted organ increases risk of cirrhosis. But use of antiviral combination therapy within the first year after transplant may clear the virus and perhaps forestall progression of the disease in 25 percent of the cases. The other 75 percent of transplant recipients can expect the disease to progress at about the same rate as it did pretransplant or somewhat faster. The survival rate, post-transplant, is the same as for any other group of organ transplant patients: 80 percent after one year and 70 percent after five years.

Some further statistics on liver transplantation:

- The short-term survival rate for liver transplantation was 60 percent in 1980, 70 percent in 1996, and surpassed 80 percent by 1997.
- Current statistics from OPTN (Organ Procurement & Transplantation Network):
  1-year survival rates: approx. 85 percent

3-year survival rates: approx. 75 percent

5-year survival rates: approx. 71 percent

- In 2004, 17,392 were waiting for new livers, 6,169 of liver transplants were performed, available liver donors were 6,643, and 1,858 died while waiting.
- In 2005, there were 6,444 liver transplants, 7,013 available liver donors, and 1,791 died while waiting.
- As of July 7, 2006, 17,125 patients are currently waiting for a liver transplant while there are only 2,380 available liver donors.

TREATMENTS FOR COMPLICATIONS

Encephalopathy

When liver disease leads to cirrhosis and makes it difficult for the body to clear toxins from the blood, elevated ammonia levels as well as eight to nine other chemicals may trigger fuzzy thinking and disorientation. A three-pronged approach to therapy—diet therapy, sodium benzoate, antibiotics, zinc supplementation, and the use of a lactose-based sugar—has proved helpful.

THERAPY

- Neomycin alters the chemistry and bacterial content of the intestines, lowering the levels of ammonia and other toxins released into the blood. If this drug is taken for six months or longer, hearing loss may result. Regular hearing tests are recommended, especially if you are also taking a diuretic drug called furosemide (Lasix). This medication is rarely used for encephalopathy treatment.
- Metronidazole—brand name, Flagyl—alters bacteria in the colon and intestines and may help reduce ammonia levels in the blood. The negative side effects, however, are sometimes strong: If combined with alcohol you can become very ill and sometimes there are neurological complications such as confusion and peripheral tingling or numbness.
- Rifaximin is a new medication, which is a nonabsorbable antibiotic that improves patients' mental function, probably due to changes in ammonia metabolism as well as other effects. The only major side effect is cost.
- Lactulose is a nonabsorbable sugar that changes the acid level in the colon and that reduces the amount of ammonia in the blood. The side effect is that it causes diarrhea—if it triggers more than four bowel movements a day, the dose should be reduced.
- Zinc may be useful because liver disease can create a zinc deficiency, which in turn can increase the amount of ammonia in the bloodstream. Ask your doctor for dosage guidelines.

- Sodium benzoate absorbs ammonia in the gut and carries it out of the body in the stools. It also helps reduce ammonia toxins in the liver itself.

Cirrhosis

Cirrhosis may be halted by reducing the viral load with interferon, but once it has advanced to a severe stage it is much more difficult to treat and reverse.

DIETARY TREATMENT GUIDELINES

1. No-red-meat diet if there is significant encephalopathy.
2. Eighty to 120 grams of protein each day from soy and soy products, beans, legumes, or fish. If protein consumption falls below this level, loss of muscle mass occurs—a serious medical complication.
3. Low-sodium diet.
4. Low-fat diet.

Abdominal pain

Some people report they get relief of symptoms using antigas medications such as simethicone for abdominal pain.

Itching

Some people have had good luck using Actigall or Questran to control itching.

CHINESE MEDICINE TREATMENT OPTIONS
FROM MISHA RUTH COHEN, O.M.D., L.Ac.

Before we go into the specifics of using Chinese medicine to treat HCV, I want to mention the philosophy of Chinese traditional medicine, and how it is applied in our modern era to the management of hepatitis C.

Historically, Chinese traditional medicine has not identified viruses as the causes of disease. As a result, treatment goals for disharmonies associated with liver infections have not been to combat a virus, as Western medicine tries to do. Instead, in Chinese traditional medicine the goal is to alleviate symptoms and prevent further damage to the various Organ Systems and Essential Substances that are out of harmony.

This is achieved through the use of dietary therapy, acupuncture/moxibustion (the stimulation of acupuncture points using heat from burning herbs), herbal therapy, Qi Gong exercise, and meditation. This four-pronged treatment approach can reshape your inner health and your outlook on the world. When you embrace Chinese medicine, you are tapping into a wellspring of deep relaxation, of peaceful acceptance of your place in the universe, and an understanding of the interconnectedness of mind/body/spirit.

Today this time-tested approach to healing is evolving and expanding to embrace the insights and discoveries made through science. In a few areas the two streams of medical treatment are commingling with more positive results in the treatment of viral disease such as hepatitis C. For thousands of years Chinese medicine has used treatments for liver disease that have produced positive effects. Recent studies in China and elsewhere have now confirmed that certain herbal formulas can control liver inflammation and prevent scarring, even if the viral load is still high; others have demonstrated that acupuncture can relieve symptoms associated with HCV. Repeated studies of the effects of meditation and Qi Gong on immune strength confirm that it is beneficial in managing chronic infections.

In twenty-first-century Chinese medicine there is a place for Western medication and the application of Western scientific discoveries in treating disease.

They should not displace the traditional philosophical underpinning of Chinese medicine but instead should work as a complement. Because CM does not identify viruses and bacteria as the causes of disease, we embrace both approaches, relying on the latest scientific knowledge and the wisdom of the ages.

When we use acupuncture and Chinese herbs to treat HCV, we are using them for a combination of their Chinese therapeutics and their Western capabilities. The newly created herbal formulas for treating HCV (see chapter 8) consist of herbs that have the greatest effect from a Western point of view (anti-inflammatory, hepato-protective, antiviral) and have been used traditionally for treatment of CM syndromes. For example, Chinese medicine offers a practitioner a choice of several herbs that vitalize the Xue or act to Clear Heat and Clean Toxin, but we choose the one(s) that are particularly effective in managing HCV and related symptoms.

In the following sections we will be looking at contemporary ways to use traditional healing techniques. It is my hope that this will offer people with HCV a chance to take control of their healing process, to restore emotional, mental, and physical harmony, and to use Western therapies in a way that provides the maximum benefit with the fewest side effects.

Genotypes, Viral Load, and Therapy

Tests that reveal the magnitude of HCV infection—PCR, bDNA and TMA—all test for viral load, and liver enzyme tests for ALT and AST levels allow you and your doctor to evaluate the risks and benefits of drug therapy. For example, if you have a viral load of less than 2 million copies per milliliter, you have an improved chance of sustaining a positive response to combination therapy, regardless of the genotype of HCV with which you are infected. In addition, determining the genotype and your viral load helps the doctor decide how long you need to remain on interferon:

Genotypes 2 and 3 receive six months of combination interferon and ribavirin therapy. Twenty to 25 percent of people in this country with HCV have these genotypes.

Genotypes 1a and 1b receive twelve to eighteen months of monotherapy. Seventy to 80 percent of people in this country have this genotype.

8

Chinese Herbal Therapy for Hepatitis C

I was diagnosed with hepatitis C in 1994. I had been feeling awful; I was tired and slept all the time. My mental alertness was really taxed, to say the least. My liver enzymes were ten times the normal levels. Then I developed fibromyalgia. It was an incredibly difficult time in my life.

It took a couple of years to feel somewhat stronger. By then I knew I had to give myself a "lifectomy"—to make major changes if I was going to stay healthy. I did a lot of thinking and evaluated my options.

I learned a great deal from the process of trying to educate myself about the disease. I learned not to make hasty decisions that might have long-term effects on my life. For example, when it comes to making treatment decisions, I think it's important to be very deliberate about what you choose to do.

First, you want to make sure you have the best possible Western medical care. That means you need someone who is informative and who listens to you well, in addition to having the best diagnostic skills. Then, when you know you are getting good care, you need to decide if interferon or ribavirin is the best treatment option for you.

I decided not to use interferon because it seemed like swatting a fly with an elephant. I'd had HCV for maybe thirty years and had done pretty well; my chances of developing cirrhosis had been estimated at only around 10 percent. Why should I risk the side effects from the drugs?

Instead, I opted for herbal therapy and acupuncture. They have been good for me. I've been receiving treatment from Misha for eleven years now, and I've never felt better. I've cut my fat intake to less than 30 percent of my diet and have dropped thirty pounds. Add that to my changing jobs—from being a lawyer to being a grade school teacher—and my whole quality of life has improved. I am taking herbal formulas to strengthen my immune system and reduce liver inflammation. I also get an acupuncture treatment once every two weeks; at first it was every week. My liver enzymes have remained low; I don't have any complications. When Dr. Gish did a repeat liver biopsy three years ago, we found that the stage of disease had regressed from Stage I to Stage 0. I look at Chinese medicine treatments as a long-term commitment.

I have two wonderful children and am incredibly blessed with a devoted partner, and I want to be there for the ones I love. I am in amazement sometimes that I am so joyful and fairly healthy. These last few years have been like a rebirthing.

> —LAURA, mother of two children, 12 and 15 years old, who believes she's had hepatitis C for more than forty years

HERBAL THERAPY IS THE MOST WIDELY used and extensively documented form of Chinese medicine for chronic viral hepatitis. Practitioners rely on formulas that were developed as the result of vast clinical experience over thousands of years, plus newly developed herbal blends that offer even more powerful ways to remedy chronic liver disease associated with disharmonies in various Organ Systems and Essential Substances. No wonder many people with HCV find that treatment with herbal formulas offers an alternative to current Western drug therapies.

Many of the benefits of treating hepatitis C and its complications with Chinese herbal therapy have been illuminated by contemporary scientific knowledge:

- You benefit from laboratory-based insights into the biochemical actions of herbs.
- Scientific analysis of herbs helps avoid possible toxicities.
- Taking herbs along with Western drug therapy lessens the negative side effects of the drugs.
- Herbs, along with or as an alternative to drugs, can be used to protect the liver, decrease liver inflammation, and strengthen the immune system.

CURRENT TRENDS IN HERBAL THERAPY

At the International Symposium on Viral Hepatitis and AIDS held in Beijing, China, in 1991, more than one hundred papers were presented, several of which documented the positive results of CM treatments for viral hepatitis. Studies of herbal antivirals and of Xue cooling and circulating herbs supported the results of hundreds of years of practical experience. Kevin Ergil, Ph.D., reviewed the available literature and reported that there are at least fifty-five herbal formulas that may be used to treat hepatitis. Recent herbal studies in China and Australia showed positive results in treating hepatitis C using formulas similar to those used widely in clinics in the United States.

Among the recent results of studies in China, it has been demonstrated that herbal therapy boosts the effectiveness of interferon and works effectively to counter symptoms of HCV even in the presence of other serious disorders such as aplastic anemia. Herbal formulas also normalize liver enzymes and reduce viral loads.[1] (For a more complete list of Chinese studies see the Notes for this chapter.)

In the United States several practitioners have led the way in creating effective herbal formulas for treating HCV and related syndromes. Subhuti Dharmananda, Ph.D., director of Portland's Institute for Traditional Medicine, has advocated the use of bupleurum/gardenia formula. He says, "This formula is a derivative of the traditional Chaihu Qinggan Tang (Bupleurum formula for cleansing the liver; Bupleurum and Rehmannia Combination) of the Ming Dynasty. That formula includes bupleurum, peony, gardenia, forsythia, and tangkuei as essential ingredients. Astragalus and salvia are important here to address the common problem of blood stasis associated with hepatitis C." Other formulas he recommends include salvia/ligustrum tablets and eclipta tablets. "This formula is suited to those who have Liver/Kidney Yin Deficiency complicated by Stomach or Spleen weakness. Any of these formulas could be taken along with oxymatrine tablets. In place of the vitamins given in some of the Chinese clinical trials, ITM Institute for Traditional Medicine has developed two nutritional antioxidant preparations that can be utilized: Quercenol (which includes milk thistle extract, several flavonoids, and vitamins C and E) and Alpha Curcumone (which includes alpha-lipoic acid, several antioxidant vitamins, ginseng, and curcuma)."

These formulas are available only by prescription from practitioners who have access to the ITM literature regarding the formula ingredients, therapeutic actions, and potential clinical applications.

Qing Cai Zhang, L.Ac., M.D. (China), who runs a clinic in New York City, is another practitioner who has developed effective herbal protocols for hepatitis C based on traditional Chinese formulations and modern scientific insights. He says, "Anti-liver inflammation herbal treatments can prevent liver cell degeneration, necrosis, and bring ALT and AST levels down to the normal range. The following herbs are commonly used to control liver inflammation and protect liver cells: Wu Wei Zi (*Schizandrae Fructus*), Gan Cao (*Glycyrrhiza uralensis*), Shui Fei Ji (*Silybum marianum*), Ku Shen (*Sophorae Radix*), Chui Pen Cao (*Sedi sarmentosi herba*), Chai Hu (*Bupleuri Radix*). The liver protective effects of these herbs have been tested by animal models and clinically in China. Modern Chinese medicine uses the more potent and stable isolated active ingredient compounds, such as Schisandrin, Glycyrrhizin, Silymarin, Oleanolic acid, Oxymatrine, and

Saikosaponin A and D. If the liver inflammation is quite active with ALT and AST levels three times higher than the normal range, immune regulatory herbs are used to suppress autoimmune reactions . . . Combine the use of immune regulatory and microcirculation-improving herbs, and the result of normalization of the liver enzyme levels can be sustained. If there is jaundice, the yellowish colors can be cleared within about three weeks. Subjective symptoms such as fatigue, nausea, and poor appetite can be improved within three to four weeks. The dull pain in the liver area can also be relieved within a few weeks. After two or three months of taking the herbs, a biopsy will show a reduction of the inflammation. In many patients, viral load will also be reduced and will be stabilized at a low level. Since the life span of an individual liver cell is about eighteen months, the treatment should last at least for two years in order to replace all of the inflammation-damaged liver cells."

These two approaches vary in some ways from the herbal remedies that I have designed, but the herbal concepts and therapies that each of us uses are part of a historical continuum that stretches from China's ancient past into the twenty-first century. For example, we all recognize the role of Toxic Heat and syndromes such as Damp Heat, Qi and Xue Stagnation, Yin Deficiency, Qi Deficiency (especially Spleen Qi Deficiency), in the development of HCV-associated symptoms. Furthermore, we all use Chinese herbal medicines and modern scientific remedies from China and the West.

CHINESE HERBAL PROTOCOLS FOR HCV-RELATED SYNDROMES

Over the past twenty-three years, as the research and education chairperson of Quan Yin Healing Arts Center and founder of Chicken Soup Chinese Medicine Clinic in San Francisco, I have developed herbal formulas to treat HCV-related syndromes and complications. These treatments have evolved as a result of extensive clinical experience and research studies conducted with people with HIV/AIDS and coinfection with HIV and HCV.

As early as 1988, Qing Cai Zhang, M.D. (China), and I launched a six-month study of herbal formulas used to treat people with HIV/AIDS. This helped us pinpoint the usefulness of Clear Heat Clean Toxin herbs and led to the development of new formulas designed to specifically target viral illnesses. We also determined that with HIV infection the protection of the bone marrow through strengthening and vitalizing Xue was essential if the herbal formulas were to be consistently effective. This study was reported in the proceedings from a conference sponsored by the Oriental Healing Arts Institute in California.

Over the next two years at Quan Yin I began testing formulas for treating chronic viral infections and immune dysfunction. We evaluated more than six hundred participants who remained in the trial anywhere from twelve weeks to two years. And in May 1993 I was joined by Drs. Jeffrey Burack and Donald Abrams of San Francisco General Hospital's AIDS and oncology outpatient unit in a study of the efficacy of Chinese herbs in the treatment of HIV. This study, led by Dr. Burack, was presented as a poster at the International AIDS Society Conference in June 1993, and was published in the *Journal of Acquired Immune Deficiency Syndrome* and *Human Retrovirology* in August 1996.

Through these clinical trials, I was able to develop even more specific formulas for treating immune dysfunction in conjunction with chronic viral infections. The resulting formulas were Enhance, Clear Heat, Tremella American Ginseng, and Marrow Plus, which are produced by a company called Health Concerns and are available only to practitioners.

As a result of experiences with using those formulas, in 1991, Nancy Harris, M.D., and I developed a treatment protocol for persons with chronic active hepatitis B and C. This protocol has been used extensively at Quan Yin Healing Arts Center and at my private clinic. Over the past decade the protocol has produced far-reaching positive effects. It often helps normalize enzyme levels, and people report feeling better overall.

Today in my clinic I use a blend of traditional and modern formulas to treat hepatitis C and associated syndromes. These newer formulas that I have developed are designed to give practitioners more flexibility in prescribing for individual treatment needs. The development of the new formulas is based on traditional theory, current Chinese research, and the experiences of U.S. colleagues. Thanks go to Dr. Wei Bei Hai (Beijing), Dr. Subhuti Dharmananda (Portland, Oregon), the Gateway Clinic in London for their pioneering work in the area of hepatitis C and Chinese herbal medicine, as well as the many practitioners and clients who have given us feedback on the formulas and associated protocols over the years. We predominantly use Health Concerns, Plum Flower–brand herbs from Mayway Herbs, and Seven Forests for many pills; KPC Herbs for powders and extracts; and Spring Wind Herbs and Mayway for bulk herbs. I have designed several of the Health Concerns formulas, such as Cordyseng, Enhance, Clear Heat, Hepatoplex One, and Hepatoplex Two.

These are not the only effective herbal medications available. Your practitioner may offer other formulas from raw herbs that you cook at home, or you may purchase other pill formulas. However, you should always make sure that whatever you use comes from a well-trained and experienced herbalist, or a company that observes controlled, consistent manufacturing standards. Choosing safe, well-produced herbs is important. For more information on recommended sources, see Appendix I: Resources. Remember, herbs are powerful medicine and must be used under the supervision of a knowledgeable practitioner.

You should always inform your herbalist and your Western physician of any herbal formulas and drugs you are going to take or are already taking so they can be on the lookout for possible drug interactions or toxicities.

HCV HERBAL PROTOCOL

The basic herbal protocol that we use at Chicken Soup Chinese Medicine and Quan Yin to treat people with HCV includes formulas for immunomodulation, to treat general syndromes associated with HCV, and to counter Toxic Heat. For herbal contents of these formulas, see Appendix II: Herbal Formulas.

IMMUNOMODULATION: CORDYSENG, CORDYCEPS PS, ENHANCE, AND TREMELLA AMERICAN GINSENG

Cordyseng

This is the main formula that we use in my clinic as an immunomodulating formula for people with HCV. It is a very simple yet powerful Fu Zheng formula. When used in conjunction with other herbal formulas, it strengthens Qi, tonifies Yin and Yang, and strengthens the spleen, stomach, kidneys, and lungs.

SYMPTOMS ADDRESSED:

- digestive upset
- fatigue
- immune system dysfunction

CORDYSENG CONTENTS:

Cordyceps (Dong Chong Xia Cao)
Ganoderma (Ling Zhi)
Astragalus (Huang Qi)
American Ginseng (Xi Yang Shen)
Licorice (Gan Cao)
Ginger Oil Flavor

Cordyceps PS

When the main manifestation of HCV is fatigue and lethargy, we often use cordyceps alone. The herb is excellent when we want to use very few herbs and are specifically trying to improve fatigue as well as support the immune system.

CORDYCEPS PS CONTENTS:

Cordyceps fruiting body (Dong Chong Xia Cao)

Enhance

Tonifies Qi, Xue, and Jing; strengthens Marrow; strengthens Spleen/Stomach/Kidney; acts to clear Toxic Heat. Dose: twelve to twenty tablets per day.

SYMPTOMS ADDRESSED:

- immune weakness and dysfunction
- frequent colds and flu
- digestive dysfunction
- HIV/AIDS as well as HCV
- Chronic Fatigue Immune Dysfunction Syndrome (CFIDS)

Tremella American Ginseng

Can be used in two ways. With predominant Yin Deficiency it is used in place of Enhance for chronic viral disorders. With a slight Yin Deficiency it is often used as an adjunct to Enhance, Clear Heat, and Ecliptex. The formula tonifies Yin, Qi, Xue, and Jing; strengthens Marrow; strengthens spleen/stomach, Clear Heat, and toxins. Dose: twelve to twenty tablets per day.

SYMPTOMS ADDRESSED:

- immune weakness
- fatigue
- digestive and intestinal problems
- nightsweats, afternoon fevers
- Cordyseng

LIVER FORMULAS: HEPATOPLEX ONE, ECLIPTEX, AND SILYMARIN EXTRACT, 80% CONCENTRATE

Hepatoplex One

Regulates Qi, vitalizes Xue, clears Heat, and cleans Toxic Heat from the system. In order to protect digestion from cooling, this formula should be taken with other formulas that protect the Spleen and Stomach. This formula was specifically designed for the Chinese diagnoses found in hepatitis C in conjunction with modern Chinese herbal research.

To increase the effects of Tonifying Qi and Yin, this can be taken with Cordyseng.

If there is Spleen Dampness and Deficiency with loose stools, you may add Shen Ling.

If there is Liver Invading Spleen, a common scenario in chronic hepatitis, you may add Shu Gan.

For Xue Stagnation including liver fibrosis, cirrhosis, and decreased blood circulation, add Hepatoplex Two.

For Qi Stagnation with Xue Deficiency, add Woman's Balance.

For Xue Deficiency and Xue Stagnation, or to protect the bone marrow during chemotherapy or radiation, add Marrow Plus.

For chronic hepatitis you may also add the individual formulations of Licorice 25 and olive leaf extract.

For digestive problems you may also take Ginger Tabs or Quiet Digestion.

Symptoms Addressed:

- general symptoms of chronic hepatitis
- elevated liver enzyme levels

Hepatoplex One Contents:

Schizandra (Wu Wei Zi)
Astragalus (Huang Qi)
Artemesia Capillaris (Yin Chen Hao)
Forsythia
Semen Persica (Tao Ren)
Red Peony (Chi Shao)
Salvia (Dan Shen)
Citrus (Qing Pi)
Gardenia (Zhi Zi)
Buddha's Hand (Fo Shou)
Ginger (Gan Jiang)
Licorice (Gan Cao)

Ecliptex

Vitalizes Qi and Xue, tonifies Liver and Kidney Yin, and tonifies Xue. Dose: nine to twelve tablets per day.

THERAPEUTIC EFFECTS:

- Helps treat cirrhosis and resulting complications.
- Protects liver against damage from environmental chemicals, pharmaceuticals, alcohol, and other toxic agents.

WARNING:

Do not use during pregnancy.

Ecliptex was developed several years ago at Health Concerns to help protect liver function and repair hepatitis-caused liver damage. The formula is a combination of Yin tonics such as eclipta (*han lian cao*), Qi, and Xue vitalizing herbs such as salvia (*dan shen*), which, according to traditional Chinese medicine theory, helps strengthen the liver's ability to detoxify ingested substances. There are also Western herbs in the formula—including *Silybum marianum* (milk thistle), which German researchers have demonstrated protects the liver from damage. Silybum also stimulates liver cell protein synthesis by increasing the activity of ribosomal RNA, leading to more rapid recovery of liver cells after they are damaged. Leading pharmacological researcher Hildebert Wagner of Germany considers eclipta one of the most promising liver protective herbs.

Silymarin Extract, 80% Concentrate

Taken from milk thistle, a Western herb, Milk Thistle 80 is a new silymarin extract produced by Health Concerns. It is part of our basic protocol. Several other companies also produce an extract. Whatever brand you buy, make sure it is an 80 percent concentrated, standardized extract. Dose: one to four pills per day (400 to 800 milligrams). The extract is used both alone and as part of many formulas that are designed to support the liver and treat HCV-associated disorders.

In our first edition, we said that it appears to be safe for use with interferon or ribavirin. This is now unclear. There is laboratory-based evidence that milk thistle may interfere in some manner with interferon treatment. However, since this does not always translate to how an herb may interact with a drug in the human body, we cannot make a definitive statement without more evidence. While it may be controversial, Dr. Cohen recommends that milk thistle be discontinued during interferon treatment.

SYMPTOMS ADDRESSED:

- elevated liver enzymes
- fibrosis and associated liver damage

- all forms of liver inflammation
- general disorders and discomforts associated with chronic hepatitis

TOXIC HEAT FORMULA: CLEAR HEAT

Clear Heat

Clears Internal Heat and Toxins, particularly those associated with viral infections. Chinese studies indicate that some of the herbs Clear Heat contains may be antiviral. Dose: six to eighteen tablets per day.

SYMPTOMS ADDRESSED:

- fever
- fatigue
- flu-like symptoms
- digestive upset
- headaches

I developed Enhance and Clear Heat in 1990 as part of a continuing effort to establish highly effective treatment protocols for HIV and chronic viral illnesses associated with immune dysfunction. When Heat-clearing and antiviral affects are needed in conjunction with other formulas, Clear Heat can be added. There is a synergistic effect from the use of Heat-clearing herbs such as isatis, along with Fu Zheng herbs, which are designed to restore the Normal Qi, and liver-strengthening and protecting herbs. The combination may have immunomodulating effects, decrease viral load, and ease general liver inflammation.

BEYOND THE BASIC PROTOCOL

Chronic viral liver disease triggers so many complications and associated disorders that an ever-changing individual diagnosis must be made and herbal treatments must be tailored to a person's particular needs at any given time.

Many of the following are either traditional or variations on traditional formulas used to ease Damp Heat, Qi and Xue Stagnation, Damp Cold, Qi and Xue Deficiency, Yin Deficiency, and Toxic Heat with Dampness.

The ones described below come in one of four forms:

Tang tells you that the formula is a decoction. A decoction is made by boiling the herb or a combination of herbs in water, and then drinking the resulting liquid.

Wan or *Pian* is used to indicate that the formula is in the form of a pill or tablet.

San denotes the formula is in powder form.

For herbal contents of these formulas, see Appendix III: Herbal Formulas.

For Damp Heat

Yin Chen Hao Tang (Yin Chen Hao Decoction)

Is a decoction for jaundice arising from Dampness in Spleen or Liver Qi.

SYMPTOMS ADDRESSED:

- acute infectious hepatitis
- bright yellow skin and eyes
- abdominal fullness
- thirst
- head perspiration

Long Dan Xie Gan Tang (Long Dan Cao Decoction to Drain Liver)

Quells the upward flaring of Liver Fire, Dampness, and Heat in the liver and gallbladder channel.

SYMPTOMS ADDRESSED:

- acute hepatitis
- pain in the upper abdomen and rib cage
- chest pain
- bitter mouth
- constipation
- bloodshot eyes
- headache

Li Dan Pian (Regulate Gallbladder Pill)

Eases Damp Heat in the Liver and Gallbladder Organ Systems.

SYMPTOMS ADDRESSED:

- jaundice due to Damp Heat
- chronic inflammation of bile ducts
- acute or chronic inflammation of the gallbladder
- gallstones (it helps expel smaller stones)

Coptis Purge Fire (Modified Long Dan Xie Gan Tang)

Primarily used to clear Heat and toxins (see below). This formula is based on Long Dan Xie Gan Tang (see above) with coptis as the chief ingredient. It is also effective in countering Damp Heat in the liver and gallbladder.

For Qi and Xue Stagnation

Chai Hu Su Gan San (Bupleurum Powder to Spread the Liver)

Relieves Liver Qi Stagnation and eases pain by dispersing Liver Qi and Liver Xue.

SYMPTOMS ADDRESSED:

- abdominal distension
- pain and distension through the rib cage area over the liver
- fullness in the chest
- indigestion
- depression
- constipation
- belching

Dan Zhi Xiao Yao San (Rambling Powder with Moutan and Gardenia)

Regulates Liver Qi, tonifies blood, strengthens spleen, and eliminates Liver Heat.

SYMPTOMS ADDRESSED:

- chronic hepatitis
- fever
- headache
- abdominal pain
- restlessness
- bloodshot eyes

Shu Gan Li Pi Tang (Spread the Liver and Regulate the Spleen Decoction)

Commonly used for chronic hepatitis and early stage cirrhosis. It tonifies spleen, removes Dampness, regulates Liver Qi, and vitalizes Xue.

SYMPTOMS ADDRESSED:

- digestive disturbances
- chronic abdominal pain

- chronic pain under the rib cage in the area of the liver
- lack of appetite
- hard nodules in the liver

Shu Gan Wan (Spread Liver Pill)

Regulates Liver and Stomach Organ Systems, circulates Liver Qi, and relieves pain.

SYMPTOMS ADDRESSED:

- chronic and acute hepatitis
- pain under the rib cage, epigastric pain and fullness
- depression
- loss of appetite
- indigestion

WARNING:

Do not use Shu Gan Wan during pregnancy.

Shu Gan (Spread Liver Pill)

Based on Shu Gan Wan. This formula relieves pain in the Middle Burner (pain beneath the rib cage and along the side of the torso), relieves Liver Invading Spleen, and Liver Qi Stagnation.

SYMPTOMS ADDRESSED:

- nausea
- burping
- vomiting and regurgitation
- pain under the rib cage

WARNING:

Do not use Shu Gan during pregnancy.

Xiao Chai Hu Tang (Minor Bupleurum Combination)

A much-used liver protective formula that regulates Liver Qi and dispels Heat. Although bupleurum is not ever to be used in conjunction with interferon, it is safe if you are not taking Western antiviral therapy.

SYMPTOMS ADDRESSED:

- loss of appetite
- fever and chills
- fullness and choking feeling in the chest and under the rib cage
- dry throat
- bitter taste in mouth

WARNING:

Do not take with interferon or Rebetron.

Xiao Yao San (Rambling Powder)

Harmonizes liver and spleen functions, regulates Liver Qi, tonifies Xue.

SYMPTOMS ADDRESSED:

- chronic hepatitis
- loss of appetite
- pain along the sides of the torso
- lassitude
- fatigue
- headache

Woman's Balance (Bupleurum and Peony Formula)

Regulates Qi, nourishes Liver Xue and Yin, strengthens Spleen Qi, and harmonizes the Liver and Spleen Organ Systems. This is a contemporary formula based on Dan Zhi Xiao Yao San.

SYMPTOMS ADDRESSED:

- menstrual disorders such as PMS, swollen breasts, irregular periods
- mild depression
- abdominal bloating
- headaches

Wei Ling Tang (Calm the Stomach and Poria Decoction)

Used mainly for Damp Cold (see below). It may also be used for Qi and Xue Stagnation.

Channel Flow (Huo Luo Xiao Ling Dan)

A contemporary formula that regulates Qi and Xue, and warms the channels.

SYMPTOMS ADDRESSED:

- abdominal pain and cramping
- headache
- fibromyalgia

Li Gan Pian (Benefit Liver Tablets)

Clears Heat, soothes the Liver Organ System, and clears bile ducts.

SYMPTOMS ADDRESSED:

- acute hepatitis with or without jaundice
- pain in the liver area
- gallstones

GB-6 (Chuan Lian Zi)

Eases gallbladder inflammation and associated symptoms, and helps dissolve gallstones.

SYMPTOMS ADDRESSED:

- indigestion
- nausea
- pain in upper abdomen and rib cage
- gallstones

For Damp Cold

Wei Ling Tang (Calm the Stomach and Poria Decoction)

Dispels Dampness in the Spleen, regulates the flow of Qi in the Spleen and Stomach.

SYMPTOMS ADDRESSED:

- abdominal fullness
- loss of appetite
- heaviness in head and body

- watery diarrhea
- ascites

Shen Ling (Shen Ling Bai Zhu San)

Tonifies Damp Cold Spleen and drains Dampness. This is based on a traditional formula, Shen Ling Bai Zhu Wan.

Symptoms Addressed:

- loose stools and diarrhea
- lack of appetite
- fatigue
- difficulty concentrating
- fullness and bloating
- weak muscles
- anorexia

Wu Ling San (Five-Ingredient Powder with Poria)

Dispels Dampness and strengthens the Spleen Organ System.

Symptoms Addressed:

- edema
- ascites
- difficulty urinating
- vomiting after drinking water
- diarrhea

For Qi and Xue Deficiency

Ba Zhen Tang (Eight-Treasure Decoction)

Replenishes Qi and Xue.

Symptoms Addressed:

- pale or sallow face
- general fatigue
- dizziness
- shortness of breath
- loss of appetite
- anemia

Eight Treasures (Tang Kuei and Ginseng Eight)

Tonifies Qi and Xue.

SYMPTOMS ADDRESSED:

- pale or sallow face
- general fatigue
- dizziness
- shortness of breath
- loss of appetite
- anemia

Wu Ji Bai Feng Wan (Black Chicken White Phoenix Pill)

Tonifies Qi and Xue.

SYMPTOMS ADDRESSED:

- fatigue
- cold extremities
- fuzzy thinking
- poor appetite
- chronic hepatitis due to deficient Qi and Xue

Si Jun Zi Tang (Four Gentlemen Decoction)

Strengthens Qi, tonifies the Spleen and Stomach Organ Systems.

SYMPTOMS ADDRESSED:

- fatigue
- weakness
- abdominal distension
- loss of appetite
- vomiting
- diarrhea
- pale face
- soft voice

Si Wu Tang (Four Substances Decoction)

Tonifies and mildly regulates Xue.

SYMPTOMS ADDRESSED:

- abdominal pain
- pale face and lips
- dryness

Xiao Yao San (Rambling Powder)

Primarily used for Qi Stagnation and Xue Deficiency (see pages 55 and 56).

Dan Zhi Xiao Yao San (Rambling Powder with Moutan and Gardenia)

Primarily used for Qi Stagnation and Xue Deficiency with Liver Heat (see pages 55 and 56).

Woman's Balance (Bupleurum and Peony Formula)

Primarily used for Qi Stagnation and Xue Deficiency (see pages 55 and 56).

For Yin Deficiency

Yi Guan Jian (Linking Decoction)

Used when there is Yin Deficiency to replenish Yin and Jing in the Liver and Kidney; regulates the flow of Liver Qi.

SYMPTOMS ADDRESSED:

- chest and hypochondriac pain
- acid regurgitation
- dry mouth and throat
- bitter taste

For Toxic Heat with Dampness

Coptis Purge Fire (Modified Long Dan Xie Gan Tang)

Purges Fire and Toxins and dries Dampness.

SYMPTOMS ADDRESSED:

- inflammation
- urinary tract and kidney infections and dysfunctions

- skin rashes
- acute hepatitis symptoms

For Chronic Hepatitis C

Hepatoplex Two

Vitalizes Xue, increases circulation of the Xue, and improves microcirculation in the capillaries. This formula was specifically designed for the Chinese diagnoses found in hepatitis C with cirrhosis in conjunction with modern Chinese herbal research.

SYMPTOMS ADDRESSED:

- fibrosis and cirrhosis
- liver inflammation
- inflammation and enlargement of the spleen
- portal hypertension

HEPATOPLEX TWO CONTENTS:

Flos Carthami (Hong Hua)
Semen Persica (Tao Ren)
Angelica Sinensis (Dang Gui)
Ligusticum (Chuan Xiong)
Red Peony (Chi Shao)
Salvia (Dan Shen)
Fructus Auranti (Zhi Shi)
Buddha's Hand (Fo Shou)
Licorice (Gan Cao)

THE POWER OF INDIVIDUAL HERBS

Although herbal remedies are usually provided in formulas that include a constellation of herbs, it is important to look at the individual herbs that provide some of the most potent and most commonly used anti-HCV therapeutics.

Herbs that Affect Immune Functions

Herbs that regulate the immune system are called Fu Zheng herbs—literally, herbs that restore Normal Qi. They are used in China to tonify Qi and Xue, increase disease resistance, normalize various bodily functions, and regulate the immune system of people with cancer. (The herbal formulas in the HCV herbal protocol, page 96, contain Fu Zheng herbs.)

Fu Zheng herbs are often used in conjunction with what is called Jiedu/Qiuxie therapy—herbal treatments that are designed to clear toxins and Heat from the body. These herbs are very powerful and are generally used only in combination with Fu Zheng therapy, which ameliorates the potential side effects of antitoxins. Jiedu/Qiuxie herbs are traditionally used to destroy cancers and to treat Toxic Heat-related diseases, which we now know include viral and bacterial infections.

Astragalus (Huang Qi)

This is used as a tonic herb for the spleen and to augment Protective Qi (Wei Qi), which acts as the guard against Pernicious Influences. It is an important ingredient in many herbal formulas used to strengthen Qi. According to Western research, Astragalus has immune restoration capabilities in both the cell-mediated and humoral aspects of the immune system. In a Chinese study of chronic active hepatitis, the liver functions of eighteen out of thirty-one participants returned to normal. Astragalus has the ability to stimulate interferon to reduce the viral symptoms of the common cold.[2] In combination with other herbs, it helps fight infection and builds up resistance to viruses and bacteria.

Atractylodes (Bai Zhu)

Strengthens the Spleen and the Stomach Organ Systems and improves digestion; it is also used to remove Dampness. The chemical constituents include atractylone, actractylol, and vitamin A. Researchers in China have reported that Atractylodes can lower elevated blood sugar and prevent excess glycogen concentration in the liver. This herb is used in formulas to reduce swelling, ease diarrhea, treat Qi Deficiency and heart disharmonies, and enhance the immune system.

Cordyceps (Dong Chong Xia Cao)

A rare Tibetan mushroom, this is considered a tonic and supporting herb that restores energy, promotes energy, promotes longevity, and improves quality of life. In the lab it has been shown to increase natural interferon levels in animal cells. Recent controlled double-blind studies conducted in China by Christopher B. Cooper, M.D., of UCLA's medical school, demonstrated that derivatives from this mushroom can play a significant role in increasing energy and aerobic capacity. It is relatively nontoxic and is often prescribed as an additive to food. It is mainly cooked with meats in doses of 3 to 5 grams, according to Keen Chang Huang, author of *The Pharmacology of Chinese Herbs*. It is the main ingredient in the formula Cordyseng, the only ingredient in Cordyceps PS and is found in Clear Heat and in many cancer support formulas.

Ganoderma (Ling Zhi)

This is a mushroom whose active ingredients are primarily found in the spores. Traditionally, the red Ling Zhi variety is considered the most powerful. The various types contain ergosterol, coumarin, and mannitol. The herb lowers plasma cholesterol levels and can improve cardiac function. Ganoderma also contains highly active polysaccharides, which appear to have a potent immune-regulating effect. It is traditionally used to protect the liver from damage,[3] reduce the symptoms of hepatitis and lower liver enzyme levels.[4] It is the main ingredient in Enhance and is also found in Tremella American Ginseng, as well as the new formula Cordyseng.

Ginseng: American Ginseng (Xi Yang Shen) and Chinese Ginseng (Ren Shen)

American ginseng is often taken in conjunction with other herbs to nourish Yin and to tonify Qi. It is particularly useful after a fever to help counter weakness and irritability. It is found in the formulas Tremella American Ginseng and Cordyseng.

Chinese ginseng has an immunomodulating effect, according to *The Pharmacology of Chinese Herbs*, and enhances the body's resistance to many diseases. Small doses of ginseng saponins (an active chemical constituent) increase serum levels of antibodies. Chinese researchers have also found that it stimulates the production of natural interferon and increases the immune system killer cells activity. Alcohol-based ginseng extract seems to inhibit several types of cancer cell growth in lab experiments.

WARNING:

Do not use ginseng if you suffer from insomnia, high blood pressure, clotting problems, irregular heartbeat, or arrhythmia. Children should not take this herb, and pregnant women should take it only with the approval of their health-care professional.

Licorice (Gan Cao) or Licorice Root

This is the most commonly used herb in Chinese medicine formulas. In small quantities, it acts as the blending herb, which harmonizes the other herbs so that their effects can enter the channels and be transported to the Organ Systems as needed. Therapeutically, Chinese traditional medicine uses it to supplement the body, Clear Heat, regulate digestion, clear fluid from the lungs, and energize the spleen. Clinically, it may be used as a primary herb for more disorders than any other plant—coughs, stomach aches, acute respiratory problems, adrenal exhaustion, general inflammatory conditions, hormone-related gynecological problems, and skin rashes. Over the past twenty years Japanese researchers have found that it also has a beneficial effect on liver disorders. According to some Western herbalists, it is as powerful a liver protectant as milk thistle. *Gan Cao* is in Ecliptex, Licorice 25, Woman's Balance, and Clear Heat pill formulas.

Chemically, licorice's active ingredients are glycyrrhizin and glycyrrhetinic acid; the root contains from 6 to 14 percent, according to the Merck Company. These ingredients are often distilled from the licorice root to produce a potent extract called glycyrrhizin, which is most often used in the treatment of HCV and other viruses.

Glycyrrhizin has many antiviral uses. Research has demonstrated that it is effective against the hepatitis B virus; in Japan, clinical trials of its use in treating chronic active hepatitis have been so successful that it is now standard medical treatment there.[5] According to *The Pharmacology of Chinese Herbs,* it has also been found to be effective in the treatment of interferon-resistant chronic hepatitis C and gastric ulcers, and reduces capillary permeability, a problem in advanced stages of hepatitis C.

WARNING:

Licorice can cause adverse reactions in about 20 percent of those who take it, warns Dr. Qing Cai Zhang, and glycyrrhizin can be toxic. According to *The Pharmacology of Chinese Herbs,* a regular daily intake of 100 milligrams of glycyrrhizin or 50 grams of licorice root may trigger disturbances in the body's electrolyte balance, cause high blood pressure, reduce thyroid function, and produce other serious side effects. (Other researchers caution against taking 50 grams daily for six weeks or more.) They also caution that "elderly persons who are susceptible to the effects of licorice may show rapid deterioration of renal kidney function." Do not take glycyrrhizin during pregnancy or if you have hypertension, fluid retention problems or disorders, or kidney disease.

Herbs that Stabilize and Bind

The herbs in this category are used primarily for treating diarrhea, vomiting, excess sweating, or any other condition characterized by the excretion or expulsion of body fluids. In Chinese medicine many of these herbs are considered astringent and are said to draw fluids inward. They are particularly useful in treating symptoms associated with HCV such as chronic diarrhea, fever, nausea, abdominal pain, and headaches.

Schizandra Fruit (Wu Wei Zi)

This herb is categorized as an astringent, a Qi tonic, and a kidney tonic, and is good for calming the spirit and increasing memory functions. The fruit's main active ingredient is lignin. The rhizome contains other active ingredients.

Schizandra is particularly effective in treating liver disease. In a Chinese study, schizandra showed effectiveness in lowering liver enzyme levels in 72 percent of 102 patients over an average period of twenty-five days.[6]

It also acts as an astringent to the intestines. Chinese researchers have found that in an average of twenty-five days schizandra decreases liver enzyme levels (associated with liver disease) in almost three-quarters of people studied.[7] It is the first ingredient in Hepatoplex One and is also found in formulas such as Ecliptex, Tremella American Ginseng, Enhance, Schizandra Dreams, and Tian Wang Bu Xin Wang.

WARNING:

Schizandra may stimulate uterine contractions. Do not use if pregnant. It should also be avoided if you have epilepsy or peptic ulcers.

Ginkgo Leaf (Yin Guo Ye)

This may be helpful in treating HCV-related memory loss and depression. A double-blind study by Dr. Pierre LeBars, published in the *Journal of the American Medical Association* in October 1997, found ginkgo was effective in stabilizing or even improving dementia-related cognitive impairment in a third of people enrolled in the study, all of whom either had Alzheimer's or had suffered a stroke. It was most effective for those least impaired, suggesting that early treatment may be able to help slow deterioration. The active chemical seems to be an extract from the leaves of young ginkgo trees called EGb 761. This finding confirms the findings of many studies in Germany.

Ginkgo is also used as an anti-inflammatory and a vasodilator, and may be particularly helpful in HCV-related circulatory problems such as cold hands and feet and Raynaud's syndrome. It is a mild anticoagulant and should not be used by anyone with clotting problems or who is already taking anticoagulants without proper practitioner supervision.

Herbs that Are Antiviral, Antibacterial, and Antitoxin

Most of the herbs that have these functions are in the Clear Heat and Clean Toxin category and are used in China as antiviral and antibacterial agents. They are important elements in the fight against Toxic Heat and the symptoms associated with HCV.

Isatis Leaf (Da Qing Ye) and Isatis Root (Ban Lan Gen)

These are antiviral and antibacterial. Their main chemical component is indigo. Studies demonstrate that isatis is effective in treating viral hepatitis, herpes, and viral meningitis. In China isatis leaf and isatis root are frequently used to treat serious bacterial infections such as shigella, salmonella, streptococcus, and staphylococcus.[8]

Dandelion (Pu Gong Ying)

This herb has the Latin name *Taraxacum mongolium*; dandelion, the Western herb, has the Latin name *Taraxacum officinale*. Both are used for liver disease. Pu Gong Ying is used to treat Liver Heat disorders, especially when there are red, inflamed eyes and Damp Heat–related jaundice. Dandelion root is used to help boost the liver's detoxifying ability. As a tea it is a powerful diuretic. Its active ingredients are tarazasterol, taraxerol, taraxacerin, taraxacin, and vitamins A, B, and C. It has been shown to protect liver function and has strong antibacterial action and antiviral effects.

Marrow-Strengthening Herbs

These herbs tonify and vitalize—that is, circulate and regulate—the Xue.

Spantholobus (Ji Xue Teng)

Strengthens Kidney Jing as well as tonifies the Xue. Milletol is its main active ingredient. This herb is effective in managing the negative side effects of aplastic anemia and lowered white blood cell counts, which sometimes accompany hepatitis C.[9] Ji Xue Teng is found in Enhance, Tremella American Ginseng, and Marrow Plus formulas.

WARNING:

Pregnant women should not use Spantholobus because it can cause contractions.

Salvia (Dan Shen)

Invigorates the Xue and removes Xue stasis. It is traditionally used for soreness in the area of the rib cage that is associated with Qi and Xue Stagnation. According to Dr. Zhang, it can improve microcirculation and tissue texture in the liver. The *Materia Medica* cites a study, which found that when salvia was injected, it lowered serum cholesterol levels. It is found in Hepatoplex One and Hepatoplex Two formulas and is used to treat fibrosis, cirrhosis, liver pain, restlessness, irritability and insomnia, and stomach pain.

Herbs that Protect the Liver

Bupleurum (Chai Hu)

Used to raise the Spleen Qi, to treat digestive problems such as diarrhea or abdominal hernias, and to even out the flow of Liver Qi. It is useful in treating syndromes of advancing hepatitis C such as pain in the rib cage, a bitter taste in the mouth, and vomiting. The main chemical ingredients are bupleurumol, saponin, phytosterol, adonitol, angelicin, and various acids.[10] Bupleurum is used extensively because of its apparent ability to protect the liver from damage caused by inflammation. A study published in the journal *Hepatology* in January 1999 reported that in laboratory rats the use of a formula known as Sho-saiko-to (also called Xiao Chai Hu Tang, Minor Bupleurum Decoction), which contains bupleurum, pinellia tuber, scutellaria root, jujube fruit, ginseng root, glycyrrhiza root, and ginger rhizome may suppress "the production of hepatic fibrosis and . . . may have beneficial effects on hepatocellular carcinoma development in patients with chronic liver disease" Chai Hu is found in Xiao Yao San, Woman's Balance, and Yin Chen Hao Tang formulas.

CAUTIONARY NOTE:

One Japanese study[11] found a liver toxicity problem when bupleurum was used at the same time as interferon—at least when the herb is taken in the popular Japanese formula Sho-saiko-to (also known as Xiao Chai Hu Tang or Minor Bupleurum Combination). This is one of the reasons that the new formulas I have devised for treating HCV contain substitutes for this herb. There is some speculation that since the side effect caused by the bupleurum formula is the same as the one sometimes caused by interferon—lung fibrosis—there might be a similar mechanism of action.

Eclipta (Han Lian Cao)

Protects Liver and Kidney Yin. It is also known as a Cool Xue and Stop Bleeding herb—useful in fighting off the effects of Toxic Heat and the complications of HCV related to bleeding and circulatory problems. It is one of the main ingredients in Ecliptex herbal formula, which is designed to prevent the development of liver complications.

Silybum (Milk Thistle)

A Western herb that has long been used in Europe for the treatment of liver disorders.[12] Formulas such as Ecliptex, which is milk-thistle-based, are effective when used in conjunction with immune-modulating formulas, such as Enhance and Tremella American Ginseng, because chronic viral hepatitis is thought to be an immune dysfunction disorder as well as a viral disease. The main active ingredients in milk thistle are silymarin and flavolignins. The herb has been shown to stimulate liver cell proteins, leading to more rapid recovery of liver cells after they are damaged.[13] One Italian study found that it normalized liver enzyme levels. Silymarin, the extract of the plant, is the primary ingredient in Milk Thistle 80. In Chinese medicine the dried fruit called Shui Fei Ji is sometimes used; it appears to stimulate bile secretion and may act as a calcium channel blocker.

Also, see Silymarin Extract, 80% Concentrate, on page 99.

Scutellaria (Huang Qin)

Also known as Scullcap or scute, this herb is a potent antibacterial and anti-inflammatory agent that acts as a diuretic, a sedative, and an antihypertensive. Its principal chemical ingredients are baicalin, wogonin, and beta-sitosterol. In Chinese medicine it is used to Clear Heat and Drain Fire, and is used as an auxiliary herb for Damp Heat jaundice. In cases of Spleen and Stomach Deficiency it should only be used with Spleen and Stomach tonics and never for an extended period of time.

Although this herb appears on many lists of potential liver toxins, there is controversy surrounding that assertion. It appears that in patent formulas and tonics another herb, germander (*Teucrium*), is frequently substituted without any changes being made on the ingredient label. Germander is toxic and should be avoided. According to one of the leading scholars in herb toxicity, James Duke, Ph.D., who spent thirty years at the Department of Agriculture and in university teaching and research positions, "There is no evidence to indicate that Scutellaria is toxic when ingested at normal doses." As a clarification of the possible hazards, he goes on to state, "The FDA has suggested that overdose of the tincture causes confusion, convulsions, giddiness, pulsar irregularities, and twitching. There was a reported fatality in Norway—possibly Scutellaria, possibly Teucrium, a frequent adulterant."

Curcuma (Yu Jin)

This is a spice used worldwide. Therapeutically, this root has many benefits. According to *The Pharmacology of Chinese Herbs*, it contains an essential oil that has been found to stimulate contraction of the gallbladder and to increase bile secretion.

In general the herb acts as an anti-inflammatory. In folk medicine it has been used to counter blood stasis, and in Chinese medicine it promotes circulation of Qi and normalizes gallbladder function. It is used in the Ecliptex formula.

Gardenia Fruit (Zhi Zi)

Traditionally used for Damp Heat acute syndromes and jaundice. According to *The Pharmacology of Chinese Herbs*, it stimulates bile secretion and reduces plasma bilirubin levels, which are symptoms of both acute and advancing liver disease. Its active ingredients include gardenin, ardenoside, shanzhiside, usolic acid, crocin, and crocetin. It is used in Coptis Purge Fire and Long Dan Xie Gan Tang formulas.

Yin Chen Hao (Artemesia capillaris)

The shoots of this herb contain scoparone, chlorogenic acid, caffeic acid, beta capinene, and some essential oils. It is a long-standing treatment for jaundice, and it stimulates bile secretion. It has antibacterial and antiviral properties, and has been observed to lower cholesterol and blood pressure. Adverse effects include nausea, abdominal distension, and dizziness. It is used in Hepatoplex One and Li Dan Pian formulas.

Lychee Fruit or Fructus Lycii (Gou Qi Zi)

Used in Chinese formulas as a Xue tonic. It also tonifies the Yin of the Kidney and Liver Organ Systems and benefits the eyes. According to *Chinese Herbal Medicine: Materia Medica,* by Dan Bensky and Andrew Gamble, water extractions of Gou Qi Zi reduced the damage in the hepatic cells of mice after their exposure to carbon tetrachloride and hastened their recovery, as shown by liver function tests and an examination of liver tissue.

HERBAL TOXICITY

The liver is both a hearty organ—regenerating after disease and regaining full function under the most difficult circumstances—and a delicate assembly of tissue that can be severely injured when subject to harsh toxins that it cannot process or eliminate from the body. Any medication that you take, whether a prescription medication or an organic plant-derived herb, must be looked at for its potential to harm the liver.

For a more complete look at potentially toxic drugs and herbs, see Appendix III. Here we simply offer you precautionary guidelines and suggest standards for using herbal therapy.

First, you should feel confident that severe side effects from herbs are unusual. According to Subhuti Dharmananda, Ph.D., director of the Institute for Traditional Medicine in Portland, Oregon, "In Hong Kong, where the use of Chinese herbs is both widespread and unregulated, it has been shown that only 0.2 percent of the general medical admissions to the Prince of Wales Hospital were due to adverse reactions to Chinese medicine, as compared to 4.4 percent of admissions caused by Western pharmaceuticals." The *Journal of the American Medical Association Science News Update* for January 22, 1997, reported that researchers in Salt Lake City had determined that adverse drug events from doctor-prescribed medications may account for up to 140,000 deaths a year. The FDA has identified 180 voluntarily reported deaths from herbal dietary supplements in the past few years. Using data from the American Association of Poison Control Centers, National Center for Health Statistics, Journal of the American Medical Association, Centers for Disease Control, U.S. Consumer Products Safety Commission, and National Highway Traffic Safety Commission, the National Nutritional Foods Association compiled the following chart in 1994 for comparisons of annual deaths from other activities:

Adverse drug reactions	60,000 to 140,000
Automobile accidents	23,856
Food contamination	9,000
Boating accidents	1,064
Charcoal briquettes (carbon monoxide)	34
Household cleaners	24
Power tools	16
Hair dryers	10
All plants (house, etc.)	1

Are You Potentially Hypersensitive?

Although some herbs are simply liver toxic for all people, others create adverse reactions only in those who have particularly sensitive systems or individual allergies. You are potentially hypersensitive to herbal medication medications if you:

- have adverse reactions to drugs or herbs or have a number of different allergies;

- have a history of chronic skin rashes;
- have a preexisting liver condition.

This is important if you are being treated with herbs for a disease unrelated to hepatitis C but also have HCV. You must always be aware that beneficial medication for one disorder can have a negative impact on another coexisting disorder.

You should stop taking an herb or drug immediately if you develop a skin rash; experience nausea, bloating, tiredness, or aching in the area of the liver; or if your eyes or skin show yellowing or your feces show a reduction in color.

When herbs are used, it is best to introduce them a little at a time and to monitor reactions. Even though the frequency of adverse liver-toxic reactions is small, the damage to the liver can be severe, so it is always wise to proceed cautiously and to be alert to this uncommon possibility.

HOW TO SAFEGUARD YOUR LIVER'S HEALTH

Many, if not most, of the reported adverse reactions to herbal formulas can be eliminated if you follow some basic precautions:

- Take Chinese herbs only when prescribed by a licensed and trained practitioner.
- Make sure the herbs you take are specific for the current individual diagnosis you have received from your practitioner.
- Avoid all patent medicines and premixed potions, particularly if they are imported. Labeling mistakes are common, and frequently herbal substitutions are made in traditional formulas without being highlighted, so you end up taking herbs you (and the herbalist) do not know are in the preparation.

The herbs you take should be prescribed for their traditional use. Don't go "off label." According to the Institute for Traditional Medicine, "Whenever it is proposed to use herbs in novel ways, for example in the form of chemical extracts or for symptomatic treatment, then careful and thorough clinical research and monitoring must be undertaken. A similar caution should be applied to the prescribing of obscure or unusual herbs."

Herbs with known toxic potential should never be prescribed for those who are also taking Western drugs.

9

Chinese Nutritional Therapy

Nourishment depends on two powers, two essential abilities of the body/ mind. The first is an ability to receive, the second a power to transform.

—DAVERICK LEGGETT, *Recipes for Self-Healing*

HEPATITIS IS A LIVER DISEASE that threatens the body's ability to turn food into fuel as well as other essential proteins and blood products. Without essential proteins providing sufficient fuel for the system, all sorts of health problems can take root. And if you ingest unhealthy substances—whether food, drink, or drugs—you severely reduce the body's ability to protect itself from the hazards of HCV. You hamper the liver's miraculous ability to regenerate new liver cells. Fortunately, a wise approach to how and what you ingest can help your liver restore itself, and your body can stave off many of the complications associated with hepatitis, from fatigue to fuzzy thinking and cirrhosis.

Nutrition becomes a particularly important issue for those with complications of HCV—from the early onset of progressive liver disease to cirrhosis.[1] Malnutrition can become an increasing problem as the liver loses its capacity to process nutrients. When this happens, it is necessary to establish special dietary programs that supplement the body's diminishing supplies of vitamins, proteins, and carbohydrates.

That is why, whether you have had HCV for one year or for twenty, good nutrition is essential. But, unfortunately, eating well may be more easily said than done. In this fast and greasy food culture we live in, it takes a bit of willpower to transform your nutritional habits.

Nutrition is one area of your health that you can exert positive control over—something that feels pretty good when you are contending with a chronic disease for which there is no cure. If you start today to embrace a healthier selection of foods and forgo unhealthy habits, your tastes will gradually change. Those fatty foods you once enjoyed won't taste as good anymore. You'll like the feeling that comes from being free of alcohol or drugs. You'll enjoy feeling clear and strong. And you'll be doing one sure thing that will make you stay healthier longer and feel better about yourself in the process.

To help you make the transition, this chapter sets out the best nutritional advice from Western and Chinese traditions. In Chinese medicine, food contains powers that extend far beyond the Western concept of food as fuel that provides calories, carbohydrates, protein, fat, vitamins, and minerals. That is why dietary therapy is one of the four main healing techniques. The others are Qi Gong exercise and meditation, plus herbal therapy and acupuncture. Nutritional harmony is as essential to the healing process as taking herbs.

In Chinese medicine, food is understood to be transformed in the body into Xue and Grain Qi, an essential part of Normal Qi. This powerful distillation of food's powers nurtures not only the body but the mind and spirit as well. If food is eaten at sporadic intervals and is of low quality or insufficient quantity, then Qi and Xue Deficiencies may arise, causing systemic disharmonies, mental instability, and depression.

We will explore the underlying philosophy of dietary therapy, and offer diet programs and suggested recipes built on this healing approach to nutrition. Western recommendations and scientific data are also included. When you use the knowledge offered, you will be taking charge of your self-care in important and far-reaching ways.

THE BASICS OF CHINESE DIETARY THERAPY: ENERGETICS AND FLAVORS

Food contains certain forces that impact the harmony of Essential Substances and Organ Systems. The four Energetics—warmth, coolness, stimulation, and inhibition—are the therapeutic powers contained in food. The five flavors—sweet, spicy, sour, salty, and bitter—are the balancing agents.

Energetics can create internal harmony or throw the body out of kilter. In liver disease, when the body is unable to convert food into fuel as efficiently as it once did, your energetics are out of balance. A healthy diet harnesses these energetics so that one doesn't overpower the others.

Some foods—such as apples, tangerines, and eggplant—cool the metabolism and Organ Systems; other foods—such as chicken, leeks, and shrimp—warm the metabolism and Organ Systems.

Food such as cayenne pepper stimulates the flow of Qi and Xue, while food such as chicken inhibits their flow.

To create harmonious energetics in your diet:

1. Eat mostly warm foods, which sustain the digestive system.
2. Avoid eating raw foods frequently. The energy your body has to expend "cooking" the food after it is eaten is very depleting to those with viral infections.

3. Chew your food well to take the burden off the digestive system.
4. Drink minimal liquids while eating so you don't drown the digestive fires.
5. Avoid frozen and iced foods, which the body must work hard to warm up once they enter the stomach.
6. Eat pesticide and hormone-free foods when possible.
7. Eat in peaceful surroundings and concentrate on receiving the food. Do not eat while watching TV or while walking down the street.
8. Enjoy your food. Listen to what your body tells you about how you feel, what you need to eat, and how specific foods react in your system. If you do, your diet will become healthier, and you will get more pleasure from food.

Flavors also affect the harmony or disharmony of the mind/body/spirit. A little of any flavor tonifies (strengthens). A salty flavor concentrates. Sour contracts. Bitter descends. Sweet expands. Spicy disperses.

Every food has both an energetic and a flavor—for example, tofu is sweet and cool; chicken is sweet and warm. A balanced diet is generally composed of mostly sweet, warm foods; cold, spicy, bitter, salty, and sour are best eaten as accents.

Food Energetics

WARM FOODS

anchovy—sweet
basil—spicy
bay leaf—spicy
black pepper—spicy
brown sugar—sweet
butter—sweet
capers—spicy
cherry—sweet
chestnut—sweet
chicken—sweet
chicken liver—sweet
coconut milk—sweet
coriander—spicy
dill seed—spicy
fennel seed—spicy
garlic—spicy
ginger, fresh—spicy
leek—spicy
litchi—sweet & sour

mussel—salty
mustard green—spicy
mutton—sweet
nutmeg—spicy
onion—spicy
peach—sweet & sour
pine nut—sweet
rosemary—spicy
safflower—spicy
scallion—spicy & bitter
shrimp—sweet
sorghum—sweet
spearmint—spicy & sweet
squash—sweet
strawberry—sweet & sour
sweet potato—sweet
sweet rice—sweet
vinegar—sour & bitter
walnut—sweet

Hot Foods

cayenne—spicy
ginger, dried—spicy

soybean oil—spicy & sweet
trout—sour

Cool Foods

apple—sweet
banana—sweet
barley—sweet & salty
buckwheat—sweet
celery—sweet & bitter
cucumber—sweet
eggplant—sweet
gluten—sweet
lettuce—sweet & bitter
millet—sweet & salty
mushroom—sweet
pear—sweet

peppermint—spicy
radish—spicy & sweet
sesame oil—sweet
soybean—sweet
spinach—sweet
Swiss chard—sweet
tangerine—sweet & sour
tofu—sweet
watercress—spicy & sweet
wheat—sweet
wheat bran—sweet

Cold Foods

agar—sweet
asparagus—sweet & bitter
clam—salty
crab—salty
kelp—salty
mango—sweet & sour
mulberry—sweet
mung bean sprout—sweet
nori—sweet & salty

octopus—sweet & salty
persimmon—sweet
plantain—sweet
romaine lettuce—bitter
salt—salty
seaweed—salty
tomato—sweet & sour
watermelon—sweet

Neutral Foods

aduki bean—sweet & sour
alfalfa—bitter
almond—sweet
beef—sweet
beet—sweet
cabbage—sweet
carrot—sweet
cheese—sweet & sour
coconut meat—sweet
corn—sweet

pea—sweet
peanut—sweet
peanut oil—sweet
pineapple—sweet
plum—sweet & sour
pork—sweet & salty
potato—sweet
pumpkin—sweet
raspberry—sweet
rice—sweet

duck—sweet
egg (chicken)—sweet
fig—sweet
grape—sweet & sour
honey—sweet
kidney bean—sweet
milk—sweet
olive—sweet & sour
oyster—sweet & salty
papaya—sweet & bitter

rice bran—spicy & sweet
rye—bitter
sardine—sweet & salty
shark—sweet & salty
string bean—sweet
sugar (refined)—sweet
turnip—spicy & sweet
whitefish—sweet
yam—sweet

FOOD FLAVORS

SWEET

aduki bean (& sour)
almond
anchovy
beef
beet
brown sugar
butter
cabbage
carrot
cheese (& sour)
cherry
chestnut
chicken
chicken livers
coconut meat
coconut milk
corn
cucumber
duck
egg (chicken)
eggplant
fig
gluten
grape (& sour)
honey
kidney beans
lettuce (& bitter)
litchi (& sour)

mango (& sour)
milk
millet (& salty)
mulberry
mung bean sprout
mushroom
mutton
nori (& salty)
octopus (& salty)
olives (& sour)
oyster (& salty)
papaya (& bitter)
peach (& sour)
peanut
peanut oil
pear
persimmon
pineapple
pine nut
plantain
plum (& sour)
pork (& salty)
potato
pumpkin
raspberry
rice
sardines (& salty)
sesame oil

shark (& salty)   Swiss chard
shrimp   tangerine (& sour)
sorghum   tofu
soybean   tomato (& sour)
spinach   turnip (& spicy)
squash   walnut
strawberry (& sour)   watermelon
string bean   wheat
sugar (refined)   wheat bran
sweet potato   whitefish
sweet rice   yam

Spicy

basil   mustard green
bay leaf   nutmeg
black pepper   onion
caper   peppermint
cayenne   radish (& sweet)
coriander   rice bran (& sweet)
dill seed   rosemary
fennel seed   safflower
garlic   scallion (& bitter)
ginger, dried   soybean oil (& sweet)
ginger, fresh   spearmint (& sweet)
leek   watercress (& sweet)

Sour

trout
vinegar (& bitter)

Salty

clam   mussel
crab   salt
kelp   seaweed

Bitter

alfalfa   rye
romaine

Adapted from Bob Flaws and Honora Wolfe, *Prince Wen Hui's Cook: Chinese Dietary Therapy*. Boulder, Colorado: Paradigm Publications, 1985.

TAPPING INTO FOOD POWER

Using energetics and flavors to create a balanced and nutritious diet will allow you to fight disharmony. There are three ways that food contributes to your defense against disease.

Food Power 1: Building Qi

Food provides the body with what is called Grain Qi. This combines with the Qi that enters the body through breathing and with the Qi that is native to your body to form Normal Qi, which is what animates the body and gives it strength.

Toxic Heat—the primary agent of disharmony in hepatitis C—can interfere with the body's ability to absorb sufficient Grain Qi from the food you eat. When the Spleen and Stomach Organ Systems are affected by Toxic Heat and digestion becomes impaired, the body may lack sufficient supplies of Grain Qi, leading to greater Qi deficiencies and further Organ System complications.

Food Power 2: Nurturing the Spirit

The Shen is predominantly associated with the Heart Organ System. If excessively stimulating foods are eaten, then anxiety and restlessness may arise, and Heart Xue or Yin Deficiency can take hold. Some aspects of the Shen are associated with the Liver Organ System. When the Liver Qi and Liver Xue are in disharmony—as happens during liver disease—emotional upheaval, anxiety, and fear may arise. The Liver Organ System is particularly aligned with an aspect of the spiritual realm called the Hun or Ethereal Soul (unconscious mind). This is where courage and cowardice reside, and they depend on a healthy Liver Organ System to remain in balance. Healthy, well-balanced nutrition is vital for keeping the Liver Organ System and the mind/spirit in harmony.

Food Power 3: Supplying Life Essence

Chinese medicine believes that Jing, the Essential Substance that is the very essence of life, is constantly renewed by the food we take in. Without a steady supply of Jing from food, the stresses of life would consume the Jing we are born with, and we would wither and die prematurely.

THE FIVE-STEP LIVER SUPPORT DIET PROGRAM FOR CHRONIC HEPATITIS C *WITHOUT* CIRRHOSIS

When you are suffering from chronic hepatitis C, this five-step diet program gives the body a break—a time to calm down, gather its forces, and eliminate foods that are causing disharmony or discomfort. Through the elimination and slow reintroduction of various types of foods, the liver, stomach, and bowels can begin to function as a team again. Then the body can receive and transform food harmoniously, and balance Qi and the other Essential Substances.

The Liver Support Diet Program should be followed within the context of a total healing program under the supervision of a licensed practitioner. People with cirrhosis should not follow this program.

Each step of the program may take one day or up to one week. You and your practitioner can determine the duration. If a step seems inappropriate for your specific situation, please skip it and go on to the next one.

Do not use any step that may cause weight loss if you are already losing weight due to disease.

The steps are intended to help you detoxify as well as to rebuild your energy and health. If you feel weak or unable to do a step, skip it or shorten it.

Step One: Tonifying the Spleen and Stomach, and Moving Liver Qi

Limit your diet to the following foods:

- Miso broth: Miso is a fermented paste made from grains and beans. It contains bacteria that replenish the flora that may have been depleted or destroyed in the digestive tract through antibiotic or hormone use, poor diet, alcohol intake, or stress. Try using Mugi (barley) miso with some Mellow Yellow (light yellow miso) if it is summertime. Avoid Hatcho (dark) miso except when it is very cold.
- Vegetable broth and juices: carrot, celery, daikon, watercress, or beet juices. It is much easier to digest raw juice than raw vegetables, but you may want to cook the juice and make a hot broth.
- Lentil broth: This may also be used in addition to the vegetable broths. Cook the lentils, strain off the water, and drink as a soup.
- Brown rice cereal: This provides added protein and energy. You can find it in any natural foods store.

With Coinfection of HIV/HCV

All vegetables must be washed thoroughly to avoid parasites. Use a diluted bleach solution (½ teaspoon in a quart of water). Rinse off the bleach completely.

Step Two: Building the Xue

If your health makes it important to eat more grains and take in more calories every day, you may skip to Step Three if you wish. Add the following foods to your diet: steamed fresh vegetables, especially root vegetables (carrots, daikon root, burdock, beets) and green vegetables (broccoli, kale, chard).

Step Three: Balancing the Kidney and Cooling Toxic Heat

If you are feeling strong, follow Step Three guidelines by augmenting your diet with: cooked grains, including brown rice, millet, and barley; unbleached white rice or white basmati rice for gas or cramping. Avoid wheat, corn, and oats. No bread products are included in this step.

Step Four: Balancing the Spleen and Stomach

You may skip to Step Five. Add the following foods to your diet: fish and a wide selection of other grains and vegetables.

Step Five: For the Rest of Your Life

The above daily diet routine should be followed for a healthy life. You now have an unrestricted diet as long as you maintain an emphasis on low-fat vegetable proteins and complex carbohydrates, with a moderate amount of fish and meat. Remember, moderation, balance and harmony in flavors and types of foods are the keys to a healthy diet.

DIETARY RX FOR HEPATITIS C SYNDROMES

In Chinese dietary therapy there are foods that help counter specific disharmonies. Below are those that are particularly effective for stabilizing the syndromes associated with hepatitis C.

To Treat Liver/Gallbladder Damp Heat

In general your diet should be low in fatty and fried foods. Steamed and boiled vegetables and soups, plus bitter, sour, and salty foods are best. If there is only Heat and no Dampness, then fruits are appropriate.

GENERAL SYMPTOMS

Heat—fever, nausea, vomiting, and scanty dark urine.

HCV-RELATED SYMPTOMS

Jaundice and pain in the flanks.

Your diet should contain mung beans, watercress, barley, foods pickled without sugar, dandelion root, celery, alfalfa sprouts, spinach, chard, chrysanthemum tea, small amounts of seaweed, and barley with cabbage soup.

Your diet should not contain sugar, alcohol, stimulants, excess B vitamins or fried or fatty foods.

For Dampness Without Heat

Regular eating that supports the spleen helps to eliminate Damp conditions. Eat small meals throughout the day. Eat less sweet food and more bitter and pungent flavors.

Liver/Gallbladder Dampness

Your diet should contain aduki beans, dandelion greens, onions, leeks, scallions, small amounts of pineapple and papaya, mustard greens, horseradish, small amounts of low-fat meats, and rye.

Your diet should not contain raw fruit, tropical fruit, or bananas. Avoid eating fruit and starchy food together. Eliminate fried and fatty foods and beer.

To Treat Qi Deficiency

Qi Deficiency occurs when bad diet, lack of exercise, disharmonies in the mind/spirit, and respiration problems consume available Qi without replenishing it through diet or breathing. If conditions worsen, Qi Deficiency may become sinking Qi.

General Symptoms

Decreased appetite, fatigue, shortness of breath, and occasionally cold extremities and frequent urination.

HCV-Related Symptoms

Lethargy, loose stools, fatigue, weakness, bleeding (such as purpura), water retention, and swelling (edema) in the legs, and ascites.

Your diet should contain rice or barley broth, garlic, leeks, string beans, sunflower seeds, sesame seeds, and carrots. Half of the total calories should come from grains and legumes and a third from vegetables. About 15 percent should come from meat, but in order not to tax digestion or build mucus, eat only two or three ounces per serving. Five percent of total calories should come from dairy. To treat cold symptoms associated with Qi Deficiency you should eat dried ginger, cinnamon bark, and chicken's eggs. Do not take ginseng without a doctor's advice.

Your diet should not contain raw food, salads, fruit, and juice in excess.

To Treat Xue Deficiency

General Symptoms

Malnutrition, loss of blood, emotional stress, depletion of Qi, and Spleen Deficiency. It may also lead to insomnia, dry skin, dizziness, hair loss, palpitations, and blurry vision.

HCV-Related Symptoms

In advanced stages of cirrhosis and associated complications, liver enzyme levels often normalize and the liver becomes shrunken.

Your diet should contain oysters, sweet rice, liver, chicken soup, Dang Gui chicken (see recipe on page 148), eggs, and green beans. Added benefits come from foods that strengthen the Stomach and Spleen Organ Systems to promote sufficient production of Xue (rice, trout, small amounts of chicken, and chicken liver) and from foods that build Yin, which strengthens Xue (mussels, wheat germ, and millet).

Your diet should not contain raw fruit and vegetables, cold liquids, or ice.

To Treat Liver Qi Stagnation

GENERAL SYMPTOMS

General digestive disorders, not properly metabolizing fat, gas, mild nausea, gastritis, fibrocystic breasts, swelling or lumps in groin or breasts, goiter, PMS, menstrual irregularities, and headaches.

HCV-RELATED SYMPTOMS

Tenderness in rib cage, nausea, swollen liver and spleen, flatulence, bloating, increased liver enzymes, and fatigue.

Your diet should contain liver-sedating foods such as beef, chicken livers, celery, kelp, mussels, nori, plums, Amazake (a fermented rice drink), and foods that regulate or move Qi such as basil, rosemary, bay leaves, beets, black pepper, cabbage, coconut milk, garlic, ginger, leeks, peaches, and scallions.

Your diet should not contain alcohol, coffee, fatty foods, fried foods, excessively spicy foods, heavy red meat, sugar, or sweets.

To Treat Xue Stagnation

Xue Stagnation may be triggered by direct damage to the body's tissues, such as what happens when a virus causes liver cell inflammation, and by Qi Stagnation, Xue Deficiency, and Cold Obstructing Xue.

GENERAL SYMPTOMS

Sharp, stabbing pain along the side of the torso, abdominal pain with movement, dry skin and lips, thirst, susceptibility to cold extremities, and constipation.

HCV-RELATED SYMPTOMS

Liver tenderness and swelling, advanced cirrhosis, and liver cancer.

Your diet should contain turmeric, aduki beans, rice, spearmint, garlic, vinegar, scallions, leeks, ginger, chestnuts, rosemary, nutmeg, kohlrabi, and white pepper. You should also eat small amounts of chives, cayenne, eggplant, saffron, safflower, basil, brown sugar, and chestnuts.

Your diet should not contain duck, alcohol, fatty foods, and sweets. If you are cold, avoid citrus fruits and tomatoes.

To Treat Spleen Qi Deficiency

Spleen Qi Deficiency lingers throughout the course of hepatitis C, sometimes showing patterns of Dampness—which lead to intestinal problems such as diarrhea or loose stools—and Damp Cold or Damp Heat. Damp Cold is associated with water retention, puffiness, nausea, and intestinal upset. Damp Heat is associated with pain in the abdomen or along one side of the torso, a hot, heavy feeling and fever, which can all arise in advanced cirrhosis.

GENERAL SYMPTOMS:

Fatigue, abdominal tenderness, nausea/queasiness, lack of appetite, muscle weakness, and loose stool.

HCV-RELATED SYMPTOMS:

Malabsorption of nutrients leading to malnutrition; swollen abdomen and water retention, making breathing difficult; kidney dysfunction; and frequent urination.

Your diet should contain moderate amounts of cooked vegetables such as squash, carrots, potatoes, yams, rutabagas, turnips, leeks, and onions; grains such as rice and oats. Your diet should also contain a small amount of meat such as chicken, turkey, mutton, or beef. Other foods that provide much needed nutrients are fruits such as cooked peaches, cherries, strawberries, and figs; spices and condiments such as cardamom, ginger, cinnamon, nutmeg, and black pepper; custards; small amounts of honey, molasses, maple syrup, and sugar.

Your diet should not contain salsa, citrus, too much salt, excessive tofu, millet, buckwheat, milk, cheese, more than a small amount of seaweed, or excess sugar.

To Treat Spleen Qi Deficiency Associated with Damp Cold

Your diet should contain 65 percent of total calorie intake from grains or legumes. Around one-fourth of your calories should come from vegetables. Ten percent should come from red and white meat—no more than twenty-five ounces a week.

Your diet should not contain raw food, fruits, sugar, or dairy products.

To Treat Spleen Qi Deficiency Associated with Damp Heat

Your diet should contain 70 percent of calories from grains and legumes and 25 percent from cooked vegetables. Five percent of calories should come from white meat—not more than 12 ounces a week. An occasional salad is suggested.

Your diet should not contain red meat, raw vegetables, fruit juices, or dairy.

To Treat Spleen Qi Deficiency Associated with Dampness

Your diet should contain the foods suggested for Damp Heat, above, plus barley, corn, aduki beans, garlic, mushrooms, mustard greens, chicken, alfalfa, shrimp, scallions, and rye.

Your diet should not contain dairy, pork, shark meat, eggs, sardines, octopus, coconut milk, cucumber, duck, goose, seaweed, olives, soybeans, tofu, spinach, pine nuts, alcohol, salt, or sugar.

To Treat Yin Deficiency

Foods high in minerals and vitamins can nourish Yin, such as seaweeds and seafood, dairy, many vegetables and fruits, as well as small amounts of meat. Generally, sweet foods are recommended, while bitter, drying foods, and pungent, stimulating foods are to be avoided.

GENERAL SYMPTOMS

Weakness, afternoon or night fevers, hot flashes, hot palms, chest, or soles of feet, and difficulty sleeping.

HCV-RELATED SYMPTOMS

The chronic fatigue that accompanies HCV infection and the flu-like symptoms, such as fever and night sweats, which can arise from the virus's presence in the blood or from hepatitis C-related complications.

Your diet should contain vegetables and fruits of all types. Up to one-third of your diet can be fruit if you suffer from Dryness disorders. Also recommended are salads (when the spleen and stomach are not weak), dairy, pork, duck, seaweeds, nuts, aloe vera, and royal jelly.

Your diet should not contain stimulants, coffee, very hot spices, distilled alcohol, or too much red meat.

To Treat Kidney and Liver Yin Deficiency

The Kidney Organ System manages the body's fluid metabolism, which can become disturbed as a result of HCV infection.

GENERAL SYMPTOMS

Excessive dryness and lack of sufficient fluids. Eyes, nails, throat, and mouth can become parched. There may be muscle spasms, dizziness, and even a red hot temper. Your diet should restore moisture and feed the Yin.

HCV-RELATED SYMPTOMS

Hypertension and diabetes; headaches and irregular menses when the liver is also affected.

Your diet should contain barley, tofu, millet, asparagus, seaweed, fish, eggs, dairy, duck, pork, kelp, wheat grass, slippery elm, evening primrose oil, borage oil, flaxseed oil, nuts, and seeds.

Your diet should not contain coffee, very pungent spices, distilled alcohol, or too much red meat.

BASIC DIETARY GUIDELINES FROM WESTERN MEDICINE

Whether or not you follow the CM dietary therapy, you should make sure you follow the recommendations below.

Avoid Iron: Iron overload can occur when the liver is unable to clear it from the body. This can lead to additional liver damage and may reduce the body's positive response to antiviral treatment. In general, do not use iron supplements unless you have a proven iron deficiency.

Eliminate Drugs and Alcohol: Nutrition involves everything you ingest—food, liquids, drugs, and alcohol. In hepatitis the issue of drug and alcohol use is particularly urgent, since they both trigger accelerated damage to the liver and lead to life-threatening complications.

The one-two punch of hepatitis and alcohol inevitably accelerates the damage to the liver, and although the NIH recommends that those with hepatitis have no more than one drink a day, the smart move is to eliminate alcohol totally from your diet. You may think that since you already have cirrhosis you might as well keep drinking, but taking in more alcohol speeds the liver's destruction, greatly increases the chance of developing liver cancer, and eliminates the liver's opportunity to regenerate healthy new cells.

Drugs, both recreational and medicinal, can devastate the liver, especially when it is already under assault from HCV. Today, upward of 70 percent of all new HCV cases are people who use IV drugs. The drugs themselves burden the inflamed liver with extra toxins to process; they are associated with nutritional deficiencies, compounding the nutritional problems that arise from HCV, and speed the scarring process so that cirrhosis and liver cancer develop much more often. Prescription drugs are also dangerous for an inflamed liver. Please read Appendix III: Liver-Toxic Medications and Herbs.

Reduce Dietary Fat: Inflammation, fibrosis, and cirrhosis interfere with the ability of the liver and intestine to metabolize, process, and eliminate fat from the bloodstream. This can lead to elevated cholesterol and triglyceride levels, may make stools greasy, and affect digestion and appetite. Reduced fat intake is a benefit to almost everyone in our culture, whether they have HCV or not. We should all consider taking the following steps to ease the burden on our liver and to spare our heart.

- Reduce meat consumption to no more than three 3-ounce servings a day. Those who have encephalopathy should eliminate red meat altogether.
- Eat only 20 to 30 percent of your calories a day from fat. Only 10 percent of that should be from saturated fats.
- Reduce our consumption of whole dairy products and use low-fat or nonfat milk, cheese, and yogurt.
- Cook with canola and olive oil. Eliminate transfats such as the semi-solid fats found in margarine, if possible. They are almost as bad for you as the saturated fats found in butter, and they often come in products that are laced with food coloring and additives.

Balance Protein Sources: Adequate protein intake is essential to keep muscles strong and to give the body the resources it needs to heal and repair itself. However, it need not all come from animal sources. Vegetable protein is easier on the liver and essential in overcoming disturbances in mental function caused by high ammonia levels in the blood—encephalopathy.

One ounce of animal meat provides about seven grams of protein. An adult with (or at risk for) encephalopathy should take eighty to hundred grams of protein a day. Red meat should be omitted entirely from the diet. Chicken and fish can make up about 60 percent of dietary protein; the remaining 40 percent should come from plant protein.

The following chart reflects general guidelines from the American Liver Foundation of protein intake for those without cirrhosis.

Weight (pounds)	Recommended Protein (grams/ounces)
100	45–68/6–9
130	59–87/8–12
150	68–103/9.7–14
170	77–116/11–16
200	91–136/13–19

Please consult your doctor before altering your diet in any way. Malnutrition can be a problem for people with liver disease, and you want to make sure you take in sufficient protein from vegetable sources if you are limiting meat protein.

Reduce Sodium Intake: Severe fibrosis or cirrhosis can cause a decrease in the albumin levels in the blood and raise the venous pressure in the intestinal veins. This imbalance of proteins and pressures is quite dangerous since fluid balance and pressure are vital for maintaining the integrity of the blood vessels. When an imbalance occurs, a condition called ascites may develop. If you are diagnosed with ascites, you should restrict your diet to 500 milligrams of sodium or less a day if possible, and never exceed 1,000 milligrams to avoid extra water retention. Fluid restriction and diuretics are often necessary when this problem worsens.

Monitor Fluid Intake: Sufficient fluids are essential for the body to process nutrition and eliminate toxins. On average you should drink as many ounces of fluid a day as your weight divided by two. A 150-pound person should have 75 fluid ounces, or about nine 8-ounce glasses a day.

This is particularly important if you are taking interferon. It may help reduce the negative side effects.

Fluid retention problems can result from advanced liver disease, and you do not want to increase fluid buildup in the abdomen, legs, or arms. Alert your doctor at the first sign and discuss recommended fluid intake levels.

Special Cirrhosis Diet: Adults with cirrhosis need between 2,000 and 3,000 calories a day to allow the liver to regenerate. However, too much protein, especially in the form of red meat and animal protein, can increase ammonia in the blood and lead to encephalopathy. Patients should have 80 to 100 grams of protein per day, preferably in the form of vegetable protein or fish. Chicken and pork are less preferable, and beef protein is the least preferable because it is most likely to disturb mental function. Doctors must prescribe the amount of protein you can eat after careful evaluation of your particular needs and the ability of your liver to handle it. Some research indicates that a diet high in fats and low in protein and carbohydrates can increase the risk of cirrhosis through the development of fatty tissue in the liver. Since high-fat diets are known to stress the liver, it is probably a good idea to obtain protein from lower-fat sources such as skim milk, low-fat yogurt, lean white meats, nonfatty fish, and especially grains, pasta, and soy products.

Nonmeat protein, such as those found in soy, legumes, and beans, whole grains, and vegetables are a good source. Obtaining protein from these sources will lower ammonia levels and can make encephalopathy recede.

Keep sodium levels below 2,000 milligrams a day. Do not add salt to food on the plate or when cooking, and carefully read the labels on prepared foods. This may help avoid fluid retention and ascites.

FREQUENTLY ASKED QUESTIONS

Why Don't I Feel Like Eating?

HCV itself, or your drug therapy, can cause you to lose your appetite or to experience nausea and vomiting. If lack of appetite is the result of taking interferon or combination therapy, alert your doctor so you can take antinausea medication if you want to. It is safe, but you should have frequent blood tests to monitor the side effects. Medications that speed up the intestinal tract can be used, but diet adjustments should be the first choice. When problems persist, first make sure there is no evidence of an ulcer. Keep a food and diet diary, and note the foods you have difficulty tolerating (fat slows stomach emptying and can inhibit the appetite). Since cirrhosis results in a lack of coordination of the intestines and the digestive system, yoga, meditation, and biofeedback may also ease nausea and increase your appetite. You can also take Chinese remedies such as Curing Pills and ginger tablets.

What Should I Do On Days I Can't Eat Very Much?

Try to concentrate your protein intake in the food you can eat and talk to your practitioner or physician about taking liquid nutritional supplements. Always remember that you do not want to overtax the liver, and the benefits of taking a supplement must be weighed against the potential risks. Stay with foods that taste good to you. The virus itself and the medication can change your taste buds. Avoid strong-smelling, spicy, high-acid foods. If you find you feel full all the time, your liver may be inflamed or enlarged and pressing against your stomach; try eating five or six small meals a day.

Can Interferon Cause a Metallic Taste in My Mouth?

Yes, that is a common side effect and may make it difficult to eat. Talk to your doctor and try drinking protein- and calorie-rich drinks and smoothies if you can't face a big meal. To avoid nausea and the metallic taste associated with interferon, try taking the medication right before you go to sleep.

To help you determine your optimum nutritional levels of calories, protein, and nutrients, you may want to consult with a registered dietitian or nutritionist. A good place to start is the National Center for Nutrition and Dietetics Consumer Nutrition Hotline: 800-366-1655.

Nutritional Supplements

Using supplements is often a tricky business for those diagnosed with HCV. Malnourishment is a problem when the liver can no longer metabolize nutrients properly, so supplements sound as if they make sense. On the other hand, the liver doesn't need to be burdened with another pill to process. Overtaxing it can do damage.

Determining what is safe and smart for you depends entirely on the health of your liver and your overall well-being. Therefore, you must consult with a well-informed physician, practitioner, or nutritionist before taking any supplement.

Let's take a look at some common supplements and the recommended dosages for people who have not yet developed cirrhosis or other HCV-related complications.

Lactobacillus Acidophilus

This organism, found in natural yogurt, is used to promote beneficial bacterial growth in the digestive tract and to suppress yeast (candidiasis). It alleviates Dampness. The recommended dose is one-quarter to one-half teaspoon of powder three times a day between meals. This often helps many of the digestive problems that may be associated with hepatitis C. People who have taken many antibiotics or a high dose of antibiotics in the past may have very little naturally occurring lactobacillus acidophilus in the gut, which can lead to bowel disorders. Stool tests are recommended in this case, to see if there is a deficiency in lactobacillus acidophilus. In this case, your doctor may recommend a higher dose than what is recommended on the bottle. The best sources are powdered, lactose-free acidophilus such as Natren-brand Superdophilus. The acidophilus should be taken with room temperature or lukewarm water.

Multivitamin and Multimineral Supplement

According to the U.S. Department of Agriculture, two-thirds of Americans fail to get the Recommended Daily Allowance (RDA) of at least one vital nutrient. And those RDAs are fairly low. Most supplements supply doses far in excess of

RDAs, and ongoing research indicates there are benefits from higher doses of many vitamins.

B complex vitamins sometimes make people with hepatitis nauseated, so try to find a powered capsule form and always take it with food. As an alternative, we often recommend a sublingual regimen that includes B_{12}, B_6, and folic acid; Superior Source brand can be found at Trader Joe's or online at evitamins.com. In addition, the minerals in any multivitamin and multimineral supplement should include zinc, calcium, chromium, selenium and, copper. Be careful not to take high doses of trace minerals without the supervision of a trained practitioner or nutritionist. Niacin in high doses or in a long-acting form can cause a chemical hepatitis. It is best for people with hepatitis C that the formulas not include a lot of herbal substances and herbs be provided separately, unless an HCV-knowledgeable practitioner has prescribed the specific formula. Also, magnesium has a tendency to move Qi downward and so should not be taken as an additional supplement unless you are magnesium deficient. Furthermore, it is not recommended if you are Spleen Qi Deficient.

Low-Dose Carotenoids/Lycopenes

High doses of vitamin A can be liver toxic. Instead, take mixed carotenoids, the nontoxic building block of vitamin A, with lycopene. Lycopenes are found in vegetables such as tomatoes, and have been studied extensively and found to have anticarcinogenic effects. The recommended dose is 5,000 to 10,000 units per day.

Fat-Soluble Vitamins

If you have high bilirubin levels, you should have blood tests to check for levels of fat-soluble vitamins A, D, and K. If your levels are seriously low, your doctor can prescribe high-dose supplements and carefully monitor the results.

Vitamin C

Vitamin C cools Toxic Heat, but if you have developed Spleen Qi Deficiency with diarrhea or loose stools, a common syndrome associated with HCV, do not take C as a supplement. If you can tolerate it—it sometimes causes loose stools—consider taking it in powder form, dissolved in water to make a fizzing drink. Take up to bowel tolerance and then cut back. Vitamin C appears to work as an immune enhancer and an antioxidant, which fights the ravages of free radicals that have been linked with heart disease and cancer. High doses of vitamin C may cause kidney stones in those who have a predisposition to the disorder. Vitamin C can also erode tooth enamel, so it's important to rinse your mouth with clear water after you have taken powdered C. The Recommended Daily Allowance is 60 milligrams. Dr. Gish recommends one gram per day.

Vitamin E

You can take this in the dry form if you don't digest oils well. Vitamin E can help with cell-mediated immune function, skin problems, and memory loss. For people with severe bleeding disorders it is recommended to ask your physician before beginning Vitamin E intake. The recommended dose is 400 to 1,200 IUs per day.

Essential Fatty Acids

One tablespoon or 1,000 milligrams per day of wild salmon or krill oil, or organic flaxseed oil, can ease the aches, pains, and symptoms of fibromyalgia.

SAM-e

S-Adenosylmethionine is an essential building block of every cell in the body. Research has shown it to be effective in easing depression and arthritis. It has also shown that SAM-e can reverse liver damage and that decreases in SAM-e production are associated with chronic liver disease. According to Dr. Richard Brown of Columbia University, a leading researcher on SAM-e, there are two reliable brands that are widely available: Nature Made and GNC; for reduced cost, explore purchase on line through COSTCO and other outlets. Dr. Gish recommends 1,200 milligrams per day.

Testosterone

A testosterone deficiency can arise in men with chronic liver disease, especially if they have cirrhosis. Blood tests can determine the testosterone level, and if deficient, oral medications, injections, or transdermal patches can be administered to improve bone integrity as well as sexual function.

Low-Dose Estrogen Supplementation

Dr. Gish offers this as an option for postmenopausal women. Oral or transdermal estrogens are considered safe by most Western practitioners and do not cause a significant risk of liver injury, unless the patient has unusual liver tumors such as adenomas.

Iron

This supplement is not recommended, because it can be liver toxic. However, a Western physician may prescribe it to counter a diagnosed iron deficiency. This is common in people with liver disease because of the internal bleeding that can occur.

Zinc

This supplement assists wound healing, may boost the immune system, and is used to lower blood ammonia levels in people with cirrhosis and encephalopathy.

NOTE:

Only a licensed nutritionist or a trained, qualified practitioner should recommend additional supplements. It is important that you consult your physician when adding a supplement program beyond the basic supplements recommended.

HEALTHY FOODS FOR HCV

The following is by Dr. Lyn Patrick, NMD, adapted from the Hepatitis C Professional Certification Course.

Vitamin E

Most oils found in natural food stores, especially cold-pressed seed and grain oils, contain vitamin E. Suggested amount: 1200 IU daily. It is difficult to get all the vitamin E you need from your diet.

- Wheat germ oil: 150 IU/tablespoon
- Avocado: 23 IU per medium-sized whole avocado
- Cereal, whole-grain: 20–26 IU/ cup
- Almonds: 25 IU/cup
- Flaxseed oil: 17.5 IU/tablespoon

Omega-3 Oils

It is possible to get enough good omega-3 oils in your diet if you eat a lot of fish. If not, flaxseed oil is a good source (if it is fresh and unheated). Suggested amount: 4 grams daily

- Flaxseed oil: 8 grams/1 tablespoon
- Cod liver oil: 3 grams/1 tablespoon (be aware that this much cod liver oil also contains 13,600 IU vitamin A, a dose considered too high for someone with HCV)
- Whole flaxseeds: 2 grams/ 1 tablespoon (they have to be ground in a blender or coffee grinder to be edible)
- Walnuts: 2 grams/¼ cup
- Italian salad dressing (with canola or soy oil): .5 grams/1 tablespoon
- Salmon: 2–3 grams/1 serving (4 oz.)
- Herring: 2 grams/1 serving (4 oz.)
- Halibut: 1 gram/1 serving (4 oz.)

Vitamin C

It is difficult to get therapeutic levels of vitamin C in your diet unless you eat large amounts of fresh or fresh-frozen fruits and vegetables. There is a great difference in the vitamin C content of fresh foods depending on the variety and who does the testing. Suggested amount: 3,000 mgs. daily.

- Rosehip: 1,150–2,000 mg./1 cup
- Papaya: 300 mg./1 fruit
- Peaches, frozen: 235 mg./1 cup
- Red pepper, sweet: 283 mg./1 cup
- Mixed fruit, frozen (berries, peaches, grapes): 190 mg./1 cup
- Black currant: 150–255 mg./1 cup
- Grapefruit juice: 100 mg./1 cup
- Orange juice: 100 mg./1 cup
- Strawberries: 100 mg. /1 cup
- Guava: 183 mg./¾ cup
- Kiwi fruit: 98 mg./1 large-size fruit
- Mango: 60 mg./1 whole fruit
- Orange: 70 mg./1 whole fruit
- Strawberry: 60 mg/1 cup
- Tomato: 40 mg. /1 large, whole, ripe
- Grapefruit: 45 mg./½ med. fruit

Selenium

It is possible to get a therapeutic dose of selenium from diet alone. Suggested amount: 400 mcg. daily (especially for HIV/HCV coinfected individuals)

- Brazil nuts: 543 mcg./6–8 whole nuts
- Sardines: 150 mcg./1 can (canned in tomato sauce)
- Barley: 75 mcg./1 cup cooked whole grain barley
- Chicken: 86.4 mcg./1 cup cooked
- Fish (halibut, tuna, salmon, oysters, swordfish, shrimp): 52–68 mcg./3 oz. (1 small serving)

Zinc

It is possible to get enough zinc from diet alone. Suggested amount: 30 mg. daily (60 mg. if you have cirrhosis)

- Oysters: 74 mg./3 oz. fried oysters
- Cereal (Corn Flakes, Raisin Bran): 15 mg./1 cup
- Beans (canned): 14 mg./1 cup

Vitamin A

Safest in the vegetable (beta carotene or provitamin A) form, it is possible to get all the provitamin A you need from your diet. The more colorful the vegetable (green, yellow, orange, red) the more carotene. Suggested amount: 150,000 IU beta-carotene. Certain foods, like cod liver oil, can contain high levels of vitamin A (see omega-3 oils). Anything over 5,000 IU of vitamin A (not beta-carotene) is considered too much for someone with HCV to take in one day and may be toxic.

- Pumpkin: 38,000 IU/1 cup canned
- Sweet potato: 28,000 IU/1 cooked
- Carrots: 27,000 IU/1 cup cooked
- Spinach: 21,000 IU/1 cup cooked
- Collard greens: 19,500 IU/1 cup cooked
- Kale: 17,700 IU/1 cup cooked
- Red bell pepper: 7,400 IU/1 cup cooked
- Bok choy: 7,200 IU/1 cup cooked
- Cantaloupe: 5440 IU/1 cup raw
- Tomato paste: 4,000 IU/1 cup
- Papaya: 3,300 IU/1 raw fruit
- Mango: 1260 IU/1 raw fruit

Foods That Have High Antioxidant Activity

The following fruits and vegetables contain compounds called flavonoids and carotenoids that, together with the vitamins and minerals in the foods, allow them to act as antioxidants, an action that may be very beneficial in preventing the progression of HCV infection. This research was done by the United States Dept. of Agriculture (USDA). The numbers next to the foods are measurements of their antioxidant capacity.

- Prunes: 5,770
- Raisins: 2,830
- Blueberries: 2,400
- Blackberries: 2,036
- Cranberries: 1,750
- Kale: 1,770
- Strawberries: 1,540
- Spinach (raw): 1,260
- Raspberries: 1,220
- Brussel Sprouts: 980

- Plums: 949
- Alfalfa sprouts: 930
- Broccoli: 890
- Beets: 841
- Oranges: 750
- Red grapes: 739
- Red bell pepper: 713
- Cherries: 670
- Kiwi fruit: 602
- Other fruits and vegetables that have significant antioxidant activity: white grapes, onions, corn, eggplant, cauliflower, peas, white potatoes, sweet potatoes, cantaloupe.

Food to Avoid

Iron: Foods high in iron may be damaging to the liver in HCV infection. The following foods are considered high in iron and should be avoided if you have cirrhosis or elevated iron levels in your blood. Vitamins that contain iron should be avoided unless prescribed by a health-care provider. Nonmeat sources of iron are much less absorbable and not usually a problem. The following is a list of high iron foods.

- Organ meats
- Beef liver, kidneys
- Chicken giblets
- Turkey giblets
- Clams

Salt: Foods high in salt should be avoided if you have cirrhosis. High-salt foods cause water retention in the body and can increase edema (swelling of the feet, ankles, legs, arms, hands) and risk for ascites (swelling in the belly). The following are high-salt foods.

- Garlic salt, onion salt, seasoning salt
- MSG
- Soy sauce, miso

- Canned soups
- Canned vegetables and meats
- Bacon, sausage, ham, lunchmeat
- Processed cheese
- Potato chips, pretzels, popcorn
- Pickles, olives, sauerkraut

Supplementation Strategy: For an additional supplement strategy, Dr. Lyn Patrick of the Hepatitis C Caring Ambassadors Program recommends what she considers an essential combination of 1,200 IU of vitamin E, 400 mcg selenium, and 600 mg of alpha lipoic acid (ALA—from thioctic acid). She also recommends taking a combination of B vitamins along with this regime, as ALA can deplete the B-complex. For more information about her protocol please visit the Hepatitis C Caring Ambassadors online book *Choices* at www.hepcchallenge.org.

10

Recipes for a Healthy Liver

PART OF REVAMPING your nutritional habits is learning how to expand your cooking habits—or to develop some—so they include a new variety of healthful recipes you can prepare easily at home. The recipes in this chapter are especially designed to strengthen your constitution and to help keep the liver strong. They come from traditional Chinese sources, modern nutritionists, self-help groups, and people with HCV. Let these be a starting point for you to explore just how tasty healthy eating can be.

Basic Congee

Congee, or plain rice porridge, strengthens the constitution. By adding specific ingredients you can tailor the porridge to help treat certain conditions.

In a *3-quart* saucepan, cook 1 cup of rice (you can use brown rice if you do not have loose stools) in 7 to 9 cups of filtered water for 6 to 8 hours. An electric casserole such as a Crock-Pot is extremely useful for simmering congee while you are off doing other things. Yields approximately 3 cups congee.

Therapeutic Congees

Add about 1 cup of any vegetable ingredients in the following list to the basic rice recipe. When adding meat, use no more than 4 ounces. In general, add only between ¼ and ½ cup of the supplemental ingredients to the rice. Tip: When adding vegetables to congee, cook them with the rice. Chinese medicine theory states that this distributes the vegetables' Qi more evenly throughout the dish.

- Mung beans are for general detoxification and digestive soothing. Soak the beans and then rub off the hard-to-digest outer coating before adding to the rice pot.
- Aduki beans remove Dampness and benefit water retention, edema, ascites, and urine retention.
- Carrots are for indigestion.

- Chicken increases energy; for women, add Dang Gui and ginger.
- Lamb is for coldness and poor circulation, particularly when related to Raynaud's syndrome; for women add Dang Gui and ginger.
- Shan Yao (Dioscorea) builds Xue (blood) and is particularly good for cirrhosis and circulatory-related complications.
- Pickled daikon benefits digestion and Xue (blood).
- Dry ginger (Gan Jiang) makes a Spleen Tonic to help digestion, anorexia, and vomiting.
- Beef is for a weak Spleen Organ System, malnutrition, and hypoglycemia. Add red ginger to help improve digestion and absorption. This is warming for people who are cold.
- For an herbal tonic add 3 grams of Ren Shen (ginseng), 6 grams of Dang Gui (Angelica sinensis), 6 grams of Dang Shen (Codonopsis), two pieces of Hong Zao (Red Dates), 2 pieces of Sheng Jiang (Fresh Ginger), and/or 2 pieces of Huang Qi (Astragalus) to tonify the Qi and Xue, and to improve digestion. For loose stools add to the above 6 grams of Lian Zi (Lotus Seeds) and 9 grams of Fu Ling (Poria).
- Sweet rice strengthens the Stomach Organ System, tonifies Qi, aids digestion, and is a tonic for diarrhea and vomiting. Add 2 tablespoons of honey to water and then cook rice.

QI AND XUE TONICS

These recipes help strengthen the Qi and Xue and combat fatigue, coldness, intestinal problems related to Spleen Qi Deficiency, and anemia. You can take them once or twice a week.

When eating animal protein, remember that meat tends to be classified as warm or hot, and strengthens the Xue. Since hepatitis C is associated with Toxic Heat and with Heat conditions such as Damp Heat, meat should be eaten only in moderation; use it as flavoring to warm and to tonify Qi. Those with advancing cirrhosis and complications should avoid red meat altogether.

All animal protein can increase Dampness and trigger gas and bloating. Fatty meats are especially likely to cause Damp congestion. Lamb is considered the hottest of all meats and is good for Cold conditions. Chicken is a Qi and Xue tonic; it should be avoided by those with excessive Stagnant Qi. Chicken broth is well known as a Xue tonic and is often made with herbs such as Dang Gui for strengthening the Xue (see recipe below). With Spleen Qi Deficiency, small amounts of meat cooked for a long time in soups or congees is the best way to ingest meat.

In addition, try to eat hormone- and antibiotic-free meats, which are less toxic for the liver to process.

Fish is less warming than most meats, but fatty red fish (such as tuna) tend to be more warming and Damp producing, and should be eaten sparingly.

CHICKEN BROTH

Chicken broth is the base of many soups used as Xue and Qi tonics in Chinese medicine. Taken plain it serves as a Xue tonic. This is particularly helpful to people who have anemia, dryness of the skin, and fatigue. To make homemade broth, simply simmer in a 4-quart *soup* pot cut-up chicken parts or leftover chicken bones in 3 quarts water over low heat, covered, for at least 45 minutes. Boil down uncovered for 15 minutes. Strain and serve.

Chinese Ginger Chicken Soup

Remove skin from a whole 3-pound chicken. Place skinned chicken in a 10-quart pot and cover with water. Bring to a boil, then lower to a simmer. Add 5 scallions, sliced lengthwise and in half. Cut 1 fresh gingerroot in half and slice into slivers about 1/2 inch long and 1/16 inch wide. Add to the pot. Simmer the chicken, scallions, and ginger for 1 1/2 hours, covered. When finished, remove the chicken and debone. Return the chicken chunks to the pot. Add salt to taste if you wish. Makes four to six servings.

Dang Gui Chicken

This chicken soup, made with Dang Gui, is good for keeping the Essential Substances and Organ Systems in harmony, and for tonifying and regulating Xue.

You need a special covered Chinese clay pot that resembles an angel food cake or Bundt pan. These may be found in Chinatown shops and kitchen specialty stores.

Fill a regular 3-quart saucepan with water. Roll a 2-yard length of cheesecloth lengthwise into a long sausage shape and place as a collar along the rim of the saucepan. (When done, rinse for reuse.) Place the clay cooking pot on top of the cheesecloth ring, as the top of a double boiler. Place 1 medium chicken, cut up into about 10 pieces, in the clay pot. Add 20 grams of the herb Dang Gui. If you like, add ginger and root vegetables such as carrots, turnips, potatoes, onions, and parsnips. Cook over low heat for 1 to 2 hours, until the chicken is completely cooked and ample broth has accumulated in the upper pot. Salt to taste. Makes four servings; eat one to two servings a week.

San Qi Chicken

This soup will help vitalize Stagnant Xue. Prepare the recipe in exactly the same way as Dang Gui Chicken, above, but substitute 20 grams of San Qi to improve circulation.

MISO MAGIC

Miso is a paste made from fermented soybeans, which contain active bacteria beneficial to the digestive tract. It helps disperse Stagnant Qi and tonifies the kidney. Those on a salt-restricted diet or who have water retention or swelling in the abdomen, legs, or hands should avoid using highly salted miso.

Miso Soup with Sea Vegetables

1 strip kombu, hijiki, or other sea vegetable (available at many health food stores and Japanese groceries)
5 cups water
1 cup chopped chard, kale, or other greens
1/2 cup sliced carrots
5 teaspoons miso

Rinse the sea vegetable in cold water for 10 minutes. (If using arame, do not soak.) Wipe with a towel to remove excess sodium. Fill a pot with 5 cups of water. Cut the sea vegetable into small strips and add to the pot. Bring the water to a boil. Add the carrots, cover, and turn the heat to medium-low. Simmer for about 10 minutes. Remove a little broth to mix with the miso to form a puree. Place the miso in the pot and simmer for 2 or 3 minutes. (Miso should not be boiled, because it will kill the beneficial bacteria!) Add the greens and simmer for 2 more minutes. To increase the ability of miso to warm, add ginger. Makes four servings.

Miso Watercress Soup

This is a Xue tonic high in minerals, and it acts as a diuretic. In Western herbology, watercress is used as a liver tonic.

1 strip kombu that has been soaked and sliced
5 cups spring water
4 shiitake mushrooms, sliced
1/2 cup tofu cut into 1/4-inch cubes
4 teaspoons pureed mugi miso
1/2 bunch watercress

In a soup pot, place the kombu in the water and bring to a boil for 15 minutes. Add the mushrooms, lower the heat to a simmer, and cook for 10 minutes. Remove a little of the broth to puree the miso. Add the tofu to the miso puree, then add the mixture to the broth. Place a little watercress in each serving bowl. Pour the hot soup over. (This is enough to cook the watercress.) Makes four servings.

Speedy Miso Soup

1½ cups water
¼ cup arame (rinsed)
1 tablespoon pureed miso

Boil the water, then reduce heat so it simmers. Add the arame and cook for 2 minutes. Add the pureed miso. Makes one serving.

Hearty Miso Vegetable Soup

6 cups water
1 cup hijiki that has been soaked
1 teaspoon sesame oil
½ cup sliced carrots
½ cup diced daikon
½ cup cooked brown rice, barley, or beans
1 teaspoon grated ginger or garlic
6 fresh, medium-sized shiitake mushrooms, sliced
1 cup chopped greens (kale, chard, beet tops, etc.)
6 teaspoons pureed mugi miso
½ cup thinly sliced green onions for garnish

In a soup pot, bring the water to a boil. Add the hijiki and oil. Turn the heat to medium-low and simmer for 10 minutes. Add the carrots and daikon, and simmer for 3 minutes. Add the rice, barley, or beans, the ginger or garlic, and simmer for another 3 minutes. Add the mushrooms and greens. Simmer for 3 more minutes. Makes four to six servings.

Garnish with green onions and serve. Makes four servings.

Tahini-Miso Sauce

For a fat-restricted diet, here's a good sauce to use in place of gravies, butter, or cream sauces. It is particularly tasty over steamed vegetables, rice, and beans. Mugi (barley) miso will make a rich, dark brown sauce almost like gravy. Rice miso makes a lighter sauce.

½ cup miso
1½ cups hot water
1 tablespoon grated ginger
2 tablespoons chopped garlic
¾ cup tahini
pinch of cayenne pepper

Blend the miso with the water to make a puree. Combine with the remaining ingredients in a blender and puree for 1 minute. Place in a glass jar and refrigerate.

Makes about 16 ounces.

VEGETABLE PROTEIN—YIN AND JING TONICS

Vegetables pack a lot of nutritional power: In Western nutrition the fiber, antioxidants, vitamins, complex carbohydrates, and micronutrients they contain have been shown to reduce risks for some forms of cancer, to help lower cholesterol and reduce cardiovascular disease, to protect the digestive system, and to contribute in general to overall health and well-being. In Chinese medicine vegetables possess energetics that harmonize the Essential Substances and protect Organ System function.

- Dark green leafy vegetables tonify (strengthen) Xue, move Stagnant Liver Qi (regulate Qi by increasing its movement)
- Root vegetables strengthen Xue and Qi, nourish the Spleen with sweet flavor, and aid with Spleen and Lung Dampness conditions.
- Green foods such as barley greens, wheat grass, and chlorella have been used in Western natural nutritional medicine for building hemoglobin, due to the richness of chlorophylls (the substance responsible for the deep green color; it has a similar molecular structure to hemoglobin). Barley grass tends to reduce Dampness, while wheat grass is very cooling and may increase Dampness and Cold conditions; therefore, if one has loose stools or diarrhea, it would be better to choose barley greens over wheat grass juice.
- Vegetables with a lot of water content such as cucumbers are used to cool Heat, to moisten Dryness, and to tonify Yin.
- Small amounts of pickled (sour taste) vegetables tonify the Liver, so people with very Stagnant Liver Qi should avoid them; however, for those with Xue Deficiency, they are a good idea.
- Squash, pumpkins, and other orange and yellow vegetables are good tonifying vegetables for the Spleen and Stomach Organ Systems. Sweet potatoes are also spleen-tonifying vegetables. Carrots are highly tonifying to the

Spleen, have a warm quality, and are very easy to digest. They are also excellent for providing a wide range of carotenes.

- When you go to the store to buy your organic fresh vegetables, pick a rainbow of colors—yellows, oranges, greens, reds, purples—and you will get almost all nutrients, carotenes, lycopenes, vitamins, and minerals available.
- Sea vegetables such as kelp and nori tend to tonify the Yin and Xue. Seaweeds are also often used to resolve Dampness conditions such as swollen lymph nodes.

Hearty Lentil Soup

This all-purpose soup strengthens the Spleen and Stomach Organ Systems, benefits the heart and kidneys, and is helpful in countering Dampness.

1/2 cup green lentils
1 onion, chopped
3 stalks celery, chopped
1 carrot, chopped
3 tomatoes, chopped
2 cloves garlic, minced
1/2 cup chopped parsley
2 tablespoons tomato paste (optional)
2 tablespoons fresh thyme or 1 tablespoon dried
1/4 teaspoon sea salt
2 tablespoons cold pressed oil (sesame, safflower, olive)

Rinse the lentils twice. In a soup pot, bring to a boil in 2 cups of water. Lower the heat and simmer for about 1 hour. Add the onion, celery, and carrot. Stir while simmering another 10 minutes. Add the tomatoes and garlic. Simmer for another 3 minutes. Add the parsley, tomato paste, thyme, and salt. Simmer for 3 more minutes. Stir in the oil. Makes four servings.

Vegetable Medley Soup

This is a Xue tonic that boosts energy, eases constipation, and soothes dry skin. When cooked with cabbage, it nourishes the bone marrow and soothes digestion. Chinese cabbage (bok choy) is cooling and good for Damp Heat conditions.

1/2 cup chopped onions
1 clove garlic, minced
3 cups vegetable stock or broth
1 cup sliced carrots

½ cup chopped green beans
½ cup diced zucchini
1 cup chopped celery
2 cups slivered Swiss chard or green cabbage
½ teaspoon dried oregano
½ teaspoon dried thyme
1 cup cooked beans (kidney, lima, aduki)
1 cup chopped parsley
1 cup chopped tomatoes
½ teaspoon sea salt or strip of kombu seaweed
2 tablespoons sesame oil

In a soup pot, sauté the onions and garlic in a little oil until soft. Add the stock and bring to a boil. Add the carrots and green beans. Lower the heat and simmer for 2 or 3 minutes. Add the zucchini and celery. Simmer for another 2 minutes. Add the Swiss chard and herbs. Simmer for 3 more minutes. Add the beans, parsley, tomatoes, salt, and oil. Simmer for another 3 minutes. Makes two to four servings.

Lycopene Two-Tone Tomato Soup

Lycopene is one of the carotenes. This antioxidant is in abundant supply in this colorful soup.

1 medium onion, peeled and coarsely chopped
1 cup thinly sliced fennel bulb
3 cloves garlic, minced
2 to 3 tablespoons extra-virgin olive oil
2 tablespoons balsamic vinegar
2 pounds ripe yellow and red tomatoes, seeded, skinned, and chopped
1 cup thinly sliced fresh basil
2 tablespoons chopped fresh oregano, marjoram, or mint
salt and freshly ground pepper to taste

In a medium to large soup pot, cook the onion, fennel, and garlic in the oil until softened. Add the vinegar and cook another 5 minutes. Place the yellow and red tomatoes in separate pots. Add half of the sautéed mixture to each pot. Season with herbs. Cook for 5 minutes. Season with salt and pepper. Pour equal amounts of each color soup into bowl and swirl together. Serve hot or chilled. Makes four servings.

This recipe is from Jesse Cool, owner of the Flea Street Café in Menlo Park, California.

Kicharee

This Indian (Ayurvedic) recipe helps purify Xue, which is so important when the liver function declines.

 ½ cup mung beans or lentils, cooked
 ½ cup steamed brown rice
 1 tablespoon sesame oil or clarified butter (ghee)
 pinch of cumin seed
 ⅓ teaspoon turmeric
 1 teaspoon ground coriander
 4 cups water
 yogurt for garnish (optional)

Combine the mung beans or lentils with the rice. In a *9-inch* skillet, sauté in the oil or ghee for 5 minutes with the cumin seed, turmeric, and ground coriander. Add the water. Simmer for 20 to 25 minutes. Top with a small amount of yogurt if desired.

Hijiki Sauté

Hijiki, a Japanese seaweed, is packed with minerals and has a delicious nutlike flavor. It also tonifies the Yin, cools Heat, and moistens.

 ½ cup dry hijiki
 1 cup slivered carrots
 1 cup sliced onions
 ½ cup sliced green beans
 1 tablespoon safflower oil
 1 teaspoon grated fresh ginger
 1 tablespoon honey (optional)
 pinch of cayenne pepper
 1 teaspoon sesame oil
 1 tablespoon toasted sesame seeds

Rinse the hijiki and soak for 30 minutes. In a sauté pan, sauté the carrots, onions, and beans in the safflower oil for 3 minutes. Drain the hijiki and add to the vegetables. Sauté for 2 minutes. Add the ginger, honey if desired, and pepper. Cover and simmer for 10 minutes. Remove the cover and simmer until the excess liquid has evaporated. Remove from the heat. Add the sesame oil and seeds.

TOFU RECIPES

Soy is the main source of protein for a vast portion of the world and provides economical low-fat fuel that is easy on the digestion. It also has powerful anticancer and hormone-regulating benefits. The phytoestrogens in soy are helpful in easing the hormonal imbalances common among HCV-infected men and women. Tofu, the refined paste made from boiled, strained soybeans, is the most common way this legume is used in recipes. Although raw tofu is not recommended for people with Spleen Qi Deficiency, because it is too cold and damp, you can enjoy its many health benefits if you warm it up by frying, steaming, or sautéing it, and by adding ginger.

Soy and Thyroid

Some sources indicate that if a person has hypothyroidism—that is, low levels of thyroid hormone associated with autoimmune disease (called hashimoto's) or other causes—overconsuming soy products may damage the thyroid. But the evidence is mixed and we suggest that each person determine with his or her practitioner whether or not eating soy products may be beneficial.[1]

Tofu Toasties

1 pound firm tofu (½ inch thick)
tamari soy sauce (low-sodium if desired)
¼ cup sesame seeds

Dip the tofu in the tamari. Dip in the seeds. Toast in a toaster oven or broiler until brown. Serve with steamed or stir-fried vegetables or rice.

Instant Tofu Pesto

½ cake tofu
1 bunch green leafy vegetables, well rinsed in bleach, chopped, and lightly steamed
¼ cup olive oil
¼ cup walnut or pine nuts (optional)
several minced garlic cloves
Parmesan cheese to taste
cooked pasta

Combine all ingredients in a food processor or blender until well-mixed. Toss with cooked pasta. Serve with steamed broccoli if desired.

Peewee Pesto Pizza

Spread tofu pesto on an English muffin for a quick snack.

The above recipes are from Naomi Jay, R.N., the women's health practitioner of HIV-related research at the University of California at San Francisco, in the Departments of Stomatology and Adolescent Medicine.

Tofu Croutons

8 ounces firm tofu
1 lemon, quartered
1 quart filtered water
dash of salt

Cut the tofu into pieces
$2 \times \frac{1}{2}$ inch. Place the tofu, lemon, and water in a pot. Add the salt and boil for 15 minutes.
Remove the tofu from the water and crumble over salads, slice into vegetables or place on sandwiches.

Recipe from Carla J. Wilson, L.Ac., executive director of Quan Yin Healing Arts Center.

Grilled Tofu with Ginger

Ginger makes tofu easy to digest.

8 ounces firm tofu, sliced
1 tablespoon olive oil
1 teaspoon grated ginger

Heat the oil in a heavy frying pan. Add the ginger and sauté for 1 minute. Add the tofu slices and cook until brown on both sides and slightly crispy.
Top with Miso-Tahini Sauce (recipe below).

Recipe from Chicken Soup Chinese Medicine Clinic.

Miso-Tahini Sauce

This is a nutritious, flavorful, easy-to-digest sauce that can be added to the simplest meal. Use over grains, vegetables, or tofu.

$\frac{1}{2}$ cup tahini
$\frac{1}{2}$ cup filtered water

heaping tablespoon miso
crushed garlic or grated ginger to taste (optional)

Mix the tahini and water in a heavy saucepan. Add the miso and heat the mixture until warm but not boiling. Add more water if too thick. Add the garlic or ginger if desired.

Recipe from Chicken Soup Chinese Medicine Clinic.

Springtime Tomatillo Carrot Salsa

1 small carrot
1 large handful cilantro, finely chopped
1 to 2 cloves garlic
juice and pulp of 1 lime
1 jalapeño pepper, seeds, stems, and ribs removed
2 to 3 scallions
5 to 6 tomatillos

Combine all the ingredients in a blender or food processor. Serve with corn tortillas, as a topping for soup or as a side dish with salad.

Recipe from Beth Custer, singer/composer.

Sunflower Seed Spread

1 cup raw sunflower seeds, soaked overnight in 1/4 cup filtered water
1 1/2 tablespoons canola oil
2 tablespoons chopped fresh parsley
1 1/2 tablespoons fresh lemon juice with pulp
2 heaping teaspoons white or red miso
1 teaspoon salt substitute
1 clove garlic
1/2 teaspoon paprika
1/4 teaspoon oregano
1/4 teaspoon savory
1/4 cup chopped celery

Combine all the ingredients except the celery in a blender or food processor until well-mixed. Pour into a bowl and add the celery. Serve on rice cakes or toast or as a dip with steamed veggies.

Recipe from Beth Custer, singer/composer.

DAIRY

Dairy products tonify the Qi and Yin and are good for Dryness conditions. However, they also produce phlegm in those prone to Dampness conditions. Sheep and goat dairy tend to have a less Damp-producing quality and produce less phlegm and allergic responses.

Hormone and antibiotic-free dairy products are also a good idea to eliminate more toxins from the body and ease the burden on the liver.

FRUITS

Generally, fruits are good for countering Dryness and are cooling. People with Yin Deficiency, Excess Heat conditions and Dryness leading to constipation, Heat syndromes, mild fever, and flu-like symptoms should add raw and cooked fruit to their diet. Those diagnosed with Damp Cold conditions, in acute stages of hepatitis, or who have jaundice, bloating, abdominal pain, and loose stools, should not eat raw fruits. Cooked fruits are beneficial.

Dried fruits tend to be somewhat more warming but also tend to be sweeter and therefore more tonifying to the spleen and stomach. They should be eaten in small quantities.

Citrus fruits, such as oranges, tangerines, and grapefruits, increase Damp syndromes; however, interestingly, citrus rinds—particularly tangerine—help resolve Dampness. Tangerine peel is also used in Chinese medicine to circulate Stagnant Qi. The slightly bitter pithy white portion of the inside of the peel is filled with bioflavonoids, which are very important for those with bleeding problems and excessive bruising.

Fruit juices tend to be more cooling and purgative and should not be ingested by those with Deficient and Cold conditions.

GRAINS

Whole grains, when eaten with legumes and vegetables, provide the building blocks for protein that your body needs. When reducing the amount of animal protein you eat, be sure to increase your consumption of grains, legumes, beans, and vegetables.

In Chinese medicine, grains are the essential basis of Qi and Xue. Their sweetness nourishes the body, promoting calm and balance. They are the primary source of nourishment for the spleen, which is so severely hit by the disharmonies associated with HCV infection.

Here is a brief survey of grains, thanks to the expertise of Daverick Leggett, a world-renowned expert in Chinese nutritional therapy. These days more and more exotic forms are available, as are organic grains, offering variety and maximum benefit. Cultivate your taste buds so you can reap the rewards.

- *Rice* is a sweet food of neutral temperature that strengthens and soothes the digestive system and increases the strength of Qi and the spleen.
- *Oats* are sweet and warming, a powerful Qi tonic that can dispel Dampness and Cold. People with extreme Damp conditions should not eat oats unless they are roasted first, and they should avoid eating oats with milk or sweets, which can increase the Dampness.
- *Barley* not only nourishes Qi and Xue but it also combats Dampness and Damp Heat conditions.
- *Rye* is also good for countering Dampness, and when combined with sourdough, it helps restore balance in the presence of Liver Qi Stagnation.
- *Wheat,* the basic grain of the Western diet, triggers disharmonies and digestive problems in many people, probably because refined wheat plays far too big a role in our diet. Not only do we eat too much of it, but it offers few health benefits. And the hybrids that exist, even when eaten in wholegrain form, contain half the protein that wheat had fifty years ago. If you eat wheat, try to use organic breads, wheat germs, and sprouted wheats.
- *Buckwheat* is beneficial to the intestines and helps counter Xue Stagnation. However, those diagnosed with Wind Heat conditions should avoid it. It is also not recommended for infants or toddlers.
- *Corn* is not a complete grain: it lacks sufficient nutrients and should be eaten only with other grains that have a higher level of niacin, an essential B vitamin. It is helpful, however, in dispersing Dampness and strengthening the Kidney and Heart Organ Systems.

FLAVOR ENHANCERS

The following recipes are not for those who cannot digest fats or are on a fat-restricted diet.

Onion Butter

This can be used as a substitute for butter.

1/2 cup sesame oil
10 cups diced onions (about 4 large onions)
1 cup water
pinch of sea salt
1 teaspoon tamari sauce (optional)

Heat the oil in a 4-quart pot and sauté the onions for 10 to 12 minutes. Stir often. Add the water, salt, and tamari. Cover and bring to a boil. Lower to a simmer and cook for 4 hours, or until the onions are golden brown and very sweet. There should not be any liquid. Add more water if the onions begin to burn. Pour the onions into a blender and blend for 1 minute. Allow to cool completely. Store in a glass container in the refrigerator. Makes 1 quart.

Sesame Dressing

1/2 cup sesame butter
1 cup sesame oil
1/2 cup fresh lemon juice
1 tablespoon sea salt or tamari
1/2 chopped green bell pepper
2 stalks chopped celery
1/4 onion, chopped
1/4 cup chopped parsley or cilantro

Place all the ingredients in blender and blend until smooth. Refrigerate. Makes 3 cups.

Steaming Vegetables

When preparing a mixture of veggies, combine one root vegetable, one sea vegetable, one ground vegetable, and one leafy vegetable to keep the energetics and flavors balanced. For example:

daikon, arame, broccoli, and chard
carrot, hijiki, snow peas, and kale
beets, wakame, acorn squash, and bok choy
onions, arame, cauliflower, and mustard greens

Root vegetables may require a little longer cooking, so you can start steaming them first. Then add the lighter vegetables and the greens last. Steam the vegetables until they are cooked but still firm. Sea vegetables may need to soak in water for 10 to 15 minutes to become soft enough to steam. Rinsing after soaking will reduce the sodium level up to 50 percent.

11

Acupuncture, Moxibustion, and Acupressure

I get mad at people who think they know what I'm going through. You can't imagine how difficult hepatitis C can be—how it can wreck your life. I don't have enough energy to work full-time anymore. I don't have health insurance; I am on disability. I live alone. I wonder if life will ever be fun again.

That's what I would have told you just a few months ago, if you'd asked me about my life with hepatitis C. Today, I can tell you that I know I have a future. I can't wait to get back to work. I may even take a dance class, and I'm thinking of taking a trip to see the Cloud Forest in Costa Rica.

What accounts for this turnaround? Dramatic changes in my lifestyle: I am eating healthily; I stopped drinking any alcohol at all; and I'm taking Chinese herbs to support my immune system and help protect my liver. I also get acupuncture for my aches and pains. I have more energy than I've had in years.

—FIONA, 36, who has had hepatitis C for approximately fourteen years

THE SCIENCE AND THE ART OF HEALING do not rest solely in the hands of a doctor or practitioner. Healing is also within your grasp. As a matter of fact, without your joyful participation in the therapeutic process, there is little chance of real success. In this chapter you will discover the far-reaching therapeutic powers of acupuncture and learn how to obtain the benefits of acupressure and moxibustion at home. These therapies form a significant part of the treatment program for hepatitis C and related complications that is set out in Integrated Treatment Programs, starting on page 191 of this book.

Acupuncture—the art and science of manipulating the flow of Qi and other Essential Substances through the channels—can be used for diagnosis, treatment, and preventive medicine. By identifying areas where the Essential Substances are not flowing evenly—they may be pooled and stagnant, surging and excess, or sparse and deficient—the acupuncturist can open and close gates along the associated channels and facilitate the smooth transportation of Qi, Jing, Shen, Jin-Ye, and Xue to the Organ Systems.

Using needles, heat, and pressure, the acupuncture practitioner changes the rhythm of the substances and reestablishes harmony. This helps prevent the development of—or repairs—Organ System dysfunction associated with the inharmonious flow of Essential Substances. It is an elegant and simple system based on traditional knowledge of patterns of energy flow as it affects the Seven Emotions, Essential Substances, Organ Systems, and the channels themselves.

The Nei Jing, an ancient Chinese medicine text, identified 365 basic acupuncture points located along twelve Primary Channels, eight Extraordinary Channels, and fifteen Collaterals that are still used today. (Over the centuries more than 2,500 points have been identified, but the average practitioner uses about 150.)

DIAGNOSING HCV-RELATED SYNDROMES WITH ACUPUNCTURE

Each Organ System has a channel associated with it that supplies it with all the nourishment it needs. When a Pernicious Influence or an Epidemic Factor attacks an Organ System, the channel reflects the disharmony, alerting the practitioner to the nature of the disease or disorder. For example, when there is disharmony in the Spleen Organ System, points along the Spleen channel become tender to the touch; when Spleen 9 is tender, it may indicate that there is abnormal swelling in the abdomen, such as happens with ascites.

Preventing Development of HCV-Related Disharmony with Acupuncture

Regular use of acupuncture therapy keeps a balanced flow of the Essential Substances moving through the Organ Systems. This may strengthen the constitution so that it is better able to fight off existing disorders and prevent them from progressing. For example, Liver 14 and Gallbladder 24, which can be stimulated over the right rib cage, are used to regulate Qi and Xue, prevent stagnation, and ostensibly reduce the progression of the disease.

Treating HCV-Related Syndromes with Acupuncture

Traditional Chinese medicine acupuncture can adjust the flow of Essential Substances so that Excesses are dispersed, Deficiencies overcome, Dampness dispelled, Dryness ceased, Cold warmed, and Heat cooled. For example, Spleen 10 is a point that is worked to ease Stagnant Xue, a common syndrome associated with cirrhosis and portal hypertension.

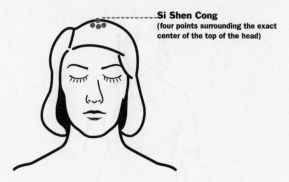

Si Shen Cong
(four points surrounding the exact
center of the top of the head)

Si Shen Cong

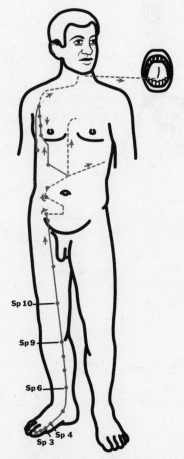

The Spleen Channel

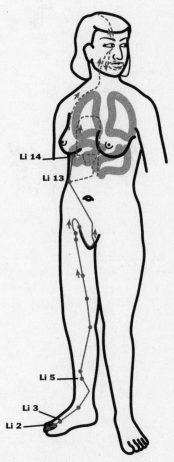

The Liver Channel

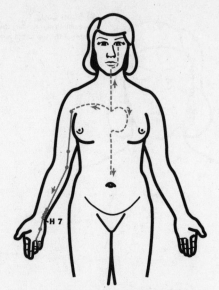

The Heart Channel

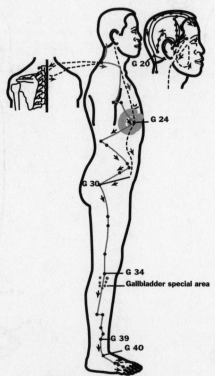

The Gallbladder Channel

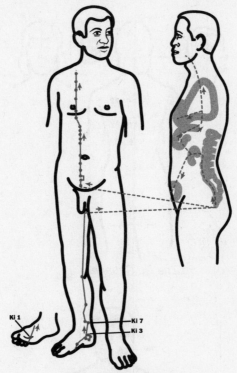

The Kidney Channel

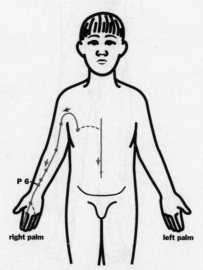

The Pericardium Channel

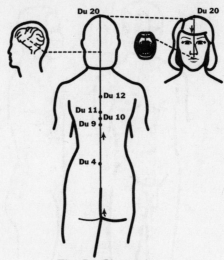

The Du Channel

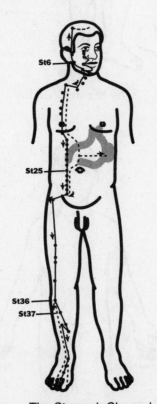

The Stomach Channel

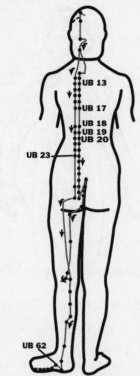

The Urinary Bladder Channel

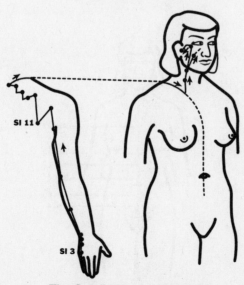

The Small Intestine Channel

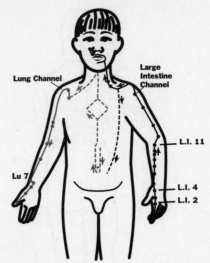

The Lung Channel and the Large Intestine Channel

Self-Acupressure Therapy

You can use acupressure to stimulate the acupoints and help ease disharmonies and strengthen the immune system.

In place of the needles, you want to apply a gentle firm touch. Using the thick, padded part of your thumb, press firmly and evenly on the area. No jabbing or poking!

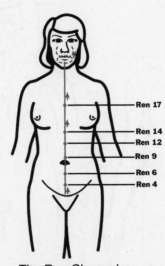

The Ren Channel

The following points are useful in treating HCV-related disorders.

For fuzzy thinking: Pericardium 6
For the brain—using reflexology point: the big toe
For depression: Ren 17 and Liver 3
For emotional disharmony: Yin Tang, the spirit point between the eyebrows.
For anxiety: Heart 7 and Pericardium 6
For headaches: Large Intestine 4 and Gallbladder 20
For stagnant blood, cirrhosis, pain, abdominal cramping, and diarrhea: Spleen 6 and 10
For ascites: Spleen 6 and 9, and a gentle abdominal massage
For nausea: Pericardium 6, Ren 12, and Spleen 4
For fatigue and weakness: Stomach 36, and Spleen 4 and 6
For abdominal cramping and digestive upset: Stomach 25 and 37
For immune system regulation: Stomach 36, Large Intestine 4, Liver 3, Lung 7, Kidney 3, and Spleen 6

WARNING:

Do not use the point Large Intestine 4 if you are pregnant.

EAR ACUPUNCTURE AND ACUPRESSURE

Ear acupuncture, also known as auriculotherapy, is highly effective for diagnosing and treating Organ System disharmony. It is also widely used by Western public health personnel to help people break and stay free of addictions to alcohol, drugs, and nicotine. In recovery centers from coast to coast, clients who are going through withdrawal from IV drugs come in for treatments on a regular basis. And best of all, a variation—ear acupressure—is a terrific tool for self-care, since it can be easily done on oneself at home.

How to massage the ear points:

Use the tip of your finger, a cotton swab, or an ear acupressure probe available at massage supply stores. Press firmly and evenly on the point. You'll know when you've hit it. The spot will be tender to the touch when there is a disharmony in the corresponding body part or Organ System.

Breathe deeply and evenly as you apply pressure. Focus on the sensation of the pressure of the ear point.

Rotate gently around the point in small circular motions. Keep the pressure firm and even. Breathe evenly.

Apply pressure to a count of ten. Release. Reapply.

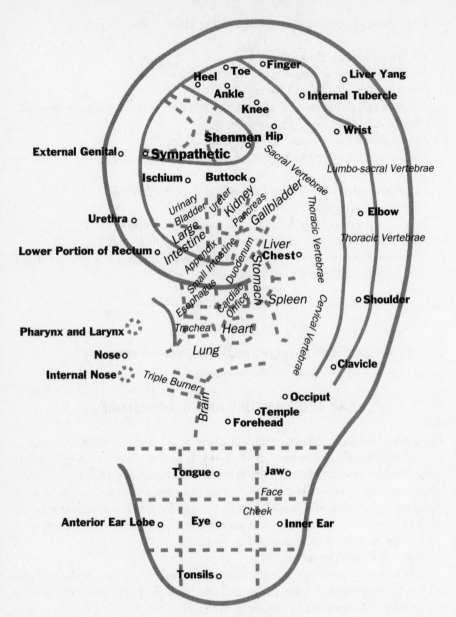

Ear Acupuncture Points

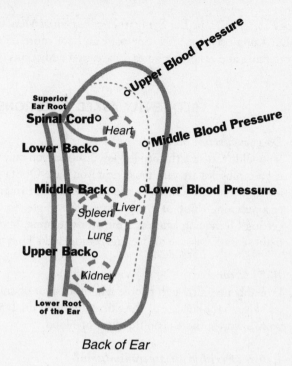

Back of Ear

If you would like to use ear acupressure on your own to treat your hepatitis-related symptoms, massaging the following points will be beneficial. (For a complete explanation of all points and their functions see Dr. Cohen's book, *The Chinese Way to Healing: Many Paths to Wholeness.*)

Spleen point: for treatment of diarrhea, chronic indigestion, and abdominal distension

Stomach point: for low fever, abdominal distension, and loss of appetite

Liver point: for Liver Qi Stagnation, irritability, gas, and fatigue that is relieved when you move around

Large Intestine point: for diarrhea and constipation

Shen Men (Spirit Gate) point: for depression and lethargy, and to ease addiction withdrawal; this provides sedation, restores peace of mind, relieves pain, and clears Heat

Heart point: for depression

Brain point: to ease fuzzy thinking and memory problems

Sympathetic point: for anxiety and stress, to ease pain

Ear Liver, Ear Kidney, Ear Spleen points: to ease Organ System disharmony associated with digestive problems, fluid retention, depression, and circulatory problems

Five Points for Detox: Ear Sympathetic, Ear Shen Men, Ear Kidney, Ear Liver, Ear Lung used together. See page 221 for more details of using ear acupuncture and other therapies for treating addictions.

FREQUENTLY ASKED QUESTIONS

Q: Does acupuncture hurt?

A: It shouldn't. When the needles are inserted, you may feel a slight sensation; if your muscles are very tense or if you have Qi Stagnation, then the feeling may intensify. Once the needles are in place you may feel nothing at all or a pulsating throb of energy or a sharp tingle. Sometimes the feeling of getting Qi moving again is a bit overwhelming, but most of the time the main sensation is one of deep relaxation and a kind of weightlessness.

Q: Will I bleed?

A: Probably not, although people who have a lot of small veins and capillaries close to the surface of the skin sometimes do. If you do, it is just a pinpoint's worth; there is no free flow of blood.

Q: Is there any risk of disease transmission?

A: Disposable sterile needles used by most practitioners these days eliminate any chance of transmission of disease.

Q: What are the risks?

A: A few cases have been reported of disease transmission and of a handful of incidents in which a doctor pierced an organ with a needle, but according to a report from Health and Human Services, "Considering the number of patients treated (estimated 9 to 12 million treatments a year) and the number of needles used per treatment (estimated average of 6 to 8), there are remarkably few serious complications."

Two cautions should be observed, however: Acupuncture can induce labor in pregnant women, and a few people may be allergic to the metals used in the needles.

Your best assurance of safety is to use a respected, experienced, licensed practitioner who practices in a professional and clean environment.

MOXIBUSTION

Moxibustion is a therapeutic technique that applies heat to acupuncture points to disperse disharmony and relieve pain. We use it in the clinic on a daily basis

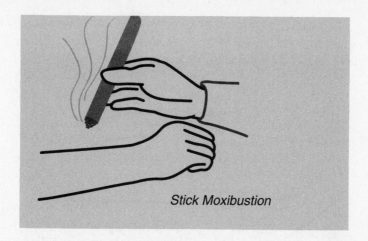

Stick Moxibustion

for all kinds of problems. Heat is generated by burning an herb—usually mugwort—molded into a cigar-shaped stick that is used as a wand held above the acupuncture point to be stimulated. The moxa sticks can be purchased from an herbalist or your practitioner. Once lit, it is held about one-and-a-half inches above the skin and the tip is moved in a circling motion above the acu-point being treated. If it is too warm, it should be moved away from the skin in half-inch intervals. It is used until you feel relaxed and can sense that the area is infused with Qi. It often helps to mark the targeted acu-point with a small dot of ink in order to keep the heat concentrated where it will do the most good.

WARNING:

Do not do self-moxibustion while lying in bed or anytime you might fall asleep. People who have severe fatigue or suffer from fuzzy thinking should ask a friend or partner for assistance.

The moxa stick burns slowly and can be used several times, so don't douse it in water or crush it out when you are through with a session; instead, seal it in an airtight jar or can until the fire is out.

You may also do moxibustion by forming the mugwort into a cone, placing it on a protective disk of the herb aconite (*Fu Zi*) or on a slice of ginger, and then setting it on a mound of salt positioned on the desired point. The cone is about one inch high and about a half inch thick and burns for three to five minutes. The most popular application is to put the aconite/moxa combo on top of a mound of salt poured into your belly button. This is particularly therapeutic if you suffer from Damp syndromes, digestive problems such as diarrhea, abdominal pains, and Cold feelings.

To use the moxa cone:

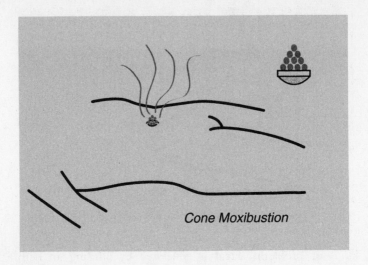

Cone Moxibustion

1. Make three cone-shaped mounds of mugwort.
2. Place each one on a slice of dry aconite or ginger (⅛ inch thick) and put within easy reach so you can retrieve them while lying down. You won't be able to sit up or move at all.
3. Place a small piece of cotton cloth nearby so you can reach it if you need to provide more insulation for your skin.
4. Lie on a firm, comfortable surface.
5. Put 2 tablespoons of salt in your navel and pat down flat. (If you have a protruding navel, Chinese texts suggest taking a long, wet noodle and forming a circle around the navel to contain the salt.)
6. Place one aconite/moxa cone on top of the salt.
7. Light the herb, not the aconite. Igniting the top of the cone assures a slower, cooler burn. Light the base, and it will burn more quickly and with more heat.
8. When the first cone burns down, replace it with the next one you prepared. When you are done with all three of them, save the aconite and brush the salt off your belly.
9. If you want to use moxibustion elsewhere on your body, substitute a cotton cloth for the salt and top it with the aconite or ginger. But be wary: Ginger isn't as good as insulation, and you can burn your skin if you're not careful.

Where to Apply Self-Moxibustion

For General HCV Treatment: Stomach 36. This is a major Qi point that tonifies and regulates Qi. It also harmonizes the Stomach and the Spleen and is good for digestive disorders and fatigue. Spleen 6 tonifies the Spleen, Kidney, and Liver. Ren 6 tonifies Deficiency and Qi.

For Dampness and Digestive Problems Associated with Cold: Ren 12.

For Lack of Appetite and Weakness: Stomach 36 and Spleen 6.

For Nausea: Ren 12 and 14, and Spleen 6.

For Ascites: Ren 6, 9, and 12, and Spleen 6 and 9.

For Cirrhosis and Associated Pain: Ren 12 and 14.

For Elevated ALT and AST Levels: You'll need a partner for these hepatitis special points that are located on the back, halfway between the inner Urinary Bladder channel and the Du channel at the level of the thoracic vertebrae 10, 11, and 12 (see illustration): Urinary Bladder 18, 19, and 20.

PRACTITIONERS' GUIDE TO ACUPUNCTURE FOR HEPATITIS

Practitioners who use traditional Chinese medicine methods are familiar with these points. These recommendations are derived from extensive clinical practice at Chicken Soup and Quan Yin clinics.

Treatment Protocol

Special points at the level of T10/T11/T12 (.75 cun from the Du channel) with moxa and needles plus UB 18, 19, 20, Yintang, and St 36 (with deficiency). Four Gates: Liver 3 and Large Intestine 4.

In addition to the basic protocol, you may want to add the following treatments for additional syndromes:

For Liver/Gallbladder Damp Heat: GB 34, Li 3, Ren 12, Sp 6, Ear-Liver, Ear-Gallbladder, P 6, Li 14, and GB 24.

For Spleen Damp Heat: Sp 9, Sp 6, Ren 12, Li 13, and P 6.

For Spleen Damp Cold: with needles and moxa Sp 9, Ren 12, P 6, St 36, and Li 13.

For Qi Stagnation: Li 3, Li 4, Ren 12, and Li 14.

For Spleen Qi Deficiency: needles and moxa St 36, Sp 3 and 6, Ren 12, P 6, and Li 13.

For Qi Deficiency: needles and moxa Ren 6, St 36, Ren 9 (moxa only), and Ki 3.

For Xue Deficiency: St 36, Sp 6, Ki 3, Ren 6, UB 17; moxa on Sp 10.

For Xue Stagnation: Ear-Sympathetic (for pain), P 6, Sp 10, L.I. 11, Li 3, Li 14, and GB 24.

Here are treatments for specific symptoms associated with hepatitis C:

Costal Pain: GB 40, Li 14, GB 24, and Li 13.

Nausea: P 6, Ren 12, and Ren 14.

Jaundice: Du 9, UB 18, and UB 19.

Diarrhea: St 36, St 37, St 25, and Ren 6.

Fatigue (due to deficiency): UB 23, St 36, Sp 6, and Ki 3.

Bleeding: Sp 10 and L.I.11. With Heat in the Xue use acupuncture only on these points; with Spleen Deficiency use moxa only on these points.

Leg Swelling: Sp 9, Sp 6, Ki 3, and Ren 6.

Ascites: Ren 9 (with moxa only).

For Detox from Addiction: Ear acupuncture on Ear Shen Men, Ear Sympathetic, Ear Lung, Ear Liver, and Ear Kidney. (See the detox program in chapter 19 for more information.)

Gallstones and Gallbladder Inflammation (Cholecystitis): GB 24; Gallbladder located about 1 cun below GB 34. (This is a floating point called simply Gallbladder; it is sensitive and activated only in the presence of gallbladder disease.)

The Effects of Acupuncture

Needling acupuncture points produces one of six effects on the Essential Substances:

1. Tonifying (or reinforcing) is used for preventive strengthening of the Organ Systems and to replenish Yin, Yang, Qi, and Xue.
2. Sedating (or reducing) dispels Heat, Cold, or Dampness, and breaks up areas of stagnation.
3. Warming is used to harmonize Essential Substances by removing blockages in the channels. This nourishes Qi, dispels Cold, and restores Yang.
4. Clearing dispels Heat, essential in countering the effects of Toxic Heat.
5. Ascending raises Qi, prevents sinking Qi, and prevents Organ System prolapse, such as a fallen bladder or uterus. This can help counter chronically loose stools.
6. Descending moves rebellious Qi downward and subdues Yang. It may be used to treat irritability and hot flashes associated with Liver Yang Rising.

12

Qi Gong: Exercise and Meditation

Careful, relaxed breathing is the foundation of most Qi Gong movements, for your breath carries with it the healing powers of well-harmonized Qi and Xue.

—LARRY WONG

RECENT STUDIES indicate that if you have symptoms or complications associated with HCV, such as portal hypertension or cirrhosis, you should avoid stressful activities. Moderate exercise is recommended, however. To start, exercise for no more than twenty minutes, three times a week. Make sure you keep your heart rate below 120 beats per minutes at all times.

For those who have less severe symptoms of HCV, it is still important to avoid overdoing it. Strenuous exercise can trigger a flare-up. When you are symptom-free, the trick is to determine, through cautious experimentation, exactly the level of exercise acceptable for you at any given time. The benefits of exercising when you can are far-reaching, and you want to do it as regularly as possible. Remember, though, that your stamina and tolerance for stress can ebb and flow over the course of this disease, sometimes quite dramatically, so if you find it difficult to exercise this month, try again next month when you have more energy and endurance.

THE QI GONG SOLUTION

Everyone knows that you live longer, look younger, and think more clearly if you get regular exercise that oxygenates the blood and tones the muscles. Add to that the emotional, physical, and spiritual benefits, and you have an essential building block of health and healing. Everyone should get as much exercise as possible, given their ability to tolerate the stress on their system. However, those who have HCV must constantly evaluate the risks of triggering a flare-up of symptoms because of overexertion. The energy-conserving, Qi-channeling practice of Qi Gong is perfectly designed to keep you in shape without causing stress and exhaustion. Furthermore, if you already have symptoms of HCV—excessive fatigue, portal hypertension, cirrhosis, or fluid retention, for example—you may have to forgo strenuous exercise altogether. Then Qi Gong meditation and breathing exercises become essential.

THE BENEFITS OF EXERCISE AND MEDITATION

Chronic illness can make you feel as if your body is beyond your control. Appropriate exercise and meditation can help you reassert your ability to shape the quality of your life and the vitality of your mind/body/spirit. Exercise and meditation assist in:

- controlling cholesterol levels and reducing fat in your body
- keeping your blood pressure low
- strengthening your cardiovascular system
- reducing stress
- reducing depression
- maintaining muscle mass
- reinforcing abstinence from alcohol and drugs
- improving and maintaining intestinal function and motility to help avoid constipation

WHAT IS QI GONG?

Qi Gong is the traditional Chinese discipline that focuses on breathing and movement of Qi to increase physical harmony and strength, and to establish spiritual and emotional peace. There are hundreds of different schools of practice; some are very vigorous—many martial arts are forms of Qi Gong—while others are extremely gentle.

Qi Gong master Larry Wong of San Francisco has designed our tour of Qi Gong. He has many students who have hepatitis C, and he shares their views on what they find most beneficial. Although you cannot learn Qi Gong from a book, I hope this series of lessons will inspire you to find a teacher or get a video (see Resources), so you can integrate these healing movements into your daily routine.

Deep Breaths

These exercises circulate Qi throughout the body, replenish depleted Qi, and calm the Shen.

The Circle of Qi

Sit on the floor cross-legged style or in a lotus position. If that is uncomfortable, you may stand up or lie down during these breathing routines.

- Inhale to a count of four to eight, depending on what you are comfortable with. There are two breathing techniques you can use: Buddha's Breath and Taoist's Breath.

For Buddha's Breath, inhale, extending your belly as you fill it up with air from the bottom of your lungs upward; exhale by pushing the air out from the bottom of your lungs first, contracting the lower rib cage and abdominal muscles, and then the upper torso. For Taoist's Breath, inhale, contracting your abdomen; exhale, letting your abdomen relax outward. You may practice these breathing techniques on alternate days.

- As you inhale, imagine the air—and your Qi—flowing evenly along the pathways of the channels.
- Become aware of the air as it enters through your nostrils and moves down the center of your chest to a spot on your abdomen about one to two inches below the navel. This is the *dan*. (Women should not concentrate on it during their periods. Concentrate on the solar plexus instead.)
- Now breathe out slowly and evenly, releasing the breath from the abdomen, up through the lungs, and out your slightly open mouth.
- As you exhale, imagine that the Qi that was at the *dan* is moving down through your pelvis, through your crotch, and up your tailbone to your lower back.
- Keep exhaling in a slow, steady, smooth stream that passes gently over your lips.
- As you inhale again, follow the Qi as it moves up along your back to your shoulders.
- Exhale and move the Qi up to the back of the head, over the top of your head, down your forehead, and returning to the nose.

At first it may be difficult to follow the flow of Qi through its cycle. Be patient and keep your breathing calm and your mind relaxed while focusing on your inhaling and exhaling.

Swing Low, Breathe Deeply

- Begin by breathing slowly and evenly. You want to feel relaxed but alert. Release your shoulders and let your arms hang loosely at your sides. Exhale and slump forward ever so slightly.

- Stand with your knees gently bent and your toes facing front.
- Gently swing your arms back and forth from the shoulders.
- Gently sway your hips as well.
- As you swing, tune in to the energy that comes up from your waist area, through your chest, and into your arms.
- Swing your arms from side to side in front of you and twist from your waist as though your torso were a damp cloth and you wanted to wring it out. (Be careful not to twist your knees or ankles; you can injure the joints.)
- Change back and forth, from swinging side to side to swinging back to front. Keep your breathing even. Clear all thoughts from your mind.
- Continue the motion for as long as you feel relaxed and comfortable but for no more than five minutes.
- When you are done, straighten up, shoulders relaxed, and continue breathing evenly and calmly.

Qi Pumping

- Stand with your toes forward and your feet shoulder's width apart.
- Gently bend your knees and begin moving up and down, keeping your feet firmly on the floor and your arms hanging limply at your sides.
- Relax your shoulders but keep your posture erect.
- Breathe into the lower part of your abdomen. Feel your lungs expand slowly. Exhale for as long as you can, releasing the air over your lips in a small, steady stream.
- Keep breathing regularly as you bounce up and down, arms flopping and shoulders relaxed, for several minutes.
- When finished, stand tall, breathing evenly. Relax.

Lion Plays with Ball

This is a sweeping motion, using one arm at a time to make a graceful arc. You will extend your hand out from the side of your body, through to the front, and then tuck it back into your waist. The power of the motion should come up from the ground, through your legs, and into your arm and torso as you inhale and exhale.

- Stand with knees relaxed. Breathe smoothly.
- Bend your arms with your elbows pointing out to the sides and your hands with fingers extended and pointing into the waist on each side of your body.
- As you inhale, extend your right arm out to the side, rotating your palm upward.

- With your arm extended, swing it around in front of you with the palm still facing upward.
- As you exhale, bend your elbow and tuck your arm against your side, bringing your hand alongside your waist. Rotate the palm downward.

Repeat using the left arm. Repeat the pair of motions ten times. You may vary the size of the circles.

Waving Hands Like Clouds

This exercise helps build and move Qi, reduces fatigue, and eases tension through the torso and spine.

- Stand with your feet at shoulder's width apart.
- Keeping your back straight, crouch forward with knees bent. You will feel your upper thigh muscles tighten.
- Place your hands, fingers extended and palms facing the floor, at waist level—one along each side of your body. The arms should be relaxed and feel light.
- Inhale slowly and gently into the bottom of your lungs.
- In a smooth motion, move your right hand across the front of your body so it is in front of your left hand.
- Slowly bring your right hand up to the level of your breastbone, rotating it so the palm is no longer facing the floor but rather perpendicular to it. Keep your left hand in its original position.
- Keeping your weight centered, exhale and smoothly rotate your body to the right. Your hands naturally follow; keep them in the same relative positions.
- Once the body is turned to the right, breathe in and slowly switch the position of your hands. Press your right hand down, moving the palm to face the floor, and lift your left arm up, moving the palm perpendicular to the floor.
- As you do this, put your legs together, knees still bent, by moving your left leg alongside the right leg.
- Exhale and turn your body to the left, letting your hands and arms follow along. Slowly repeat the cycle five times.

Zen Walking

This is one of many styles of Zen walking. It uses walking in place combined with controlled arm movements to provide many benefits. Several of the channels end in the feet and pass through the hips. By changing your posture from slumped to extended while methodically picking up and placing your feet on the floor, you massage the channels and stimulate the free flow of Qi and Xue. In addition, this exercise conditions the muscles without injuring joints or jarring tender internal organs. You may combine it with the arm-pumping exercise described below for a more vigorous routine.

Arm-Pumping Movements

- Stand in a relaxed pose, feet slightly apart, with arms hanging at the sides of the body.
- Keep your shoulders down but do not slump forward. Breathe in and out ten times in a slow, even manner. Focus on your breath. When your mind is clear and you are feeling peaceful, you are ready to begin.
- With your elbows bent and your arms at your sides, exhale as you push your flat palms down toward the floor. As you straighten out your arms, stretch your head, neck and spine up toward the ceiling. Notice your Qi flowing up.
- After a beat or two, inhale and bring your hands back up, palms still facing the floor, elbows bent. As the hands come up, hunch your shoulders. Repeat six or seven times. Inhale as your hands rise; exhale as they descend.

Walking in Place

- When you are comfortable with the previous exercise, you may combine it with a slow, intentional walk forward.
- Raise your left knee waist high and in an exaggerated motion step forward. Set your foot down on the floor very gently. Repeat the motion with your right leg. Walk forward like this for eight paces or walk in a large circle.

Combining the Arms and Legs

- As your knee rises, exhale and push your palms down toward the floor, and extend your spine, neck, and head to the ceiling. When the foot touches the ground, inhale and let your hands come back up, and hunch your back.
- Proceed in slow motion.

Wujigong's Old Dragon Washes Face

Stand with feet parallel about a shoulders' width apart, knees unlocked, hands and arms hanging loosely by your sides. This is what is known as the Wuji Posture. Tilt your pelvis slightly and hold your head high with the chin tucked in ever so slightly. (If standing is not comfortable, you may sit on a chair or your bed.)

Without touching your face, use the Lau Gong energy centers in your palms to help reduce stress. Begin by moving your hands in a wiping motion across the front of your face and down the sides below your ears. Move first the left hand, then the right, in a smooth, unforced, continuous pattern. The rotation should be from the outside to the inside (from ear to nose) with each hand. You should feel the Qi coming from your palms relaxing your upper body, cleansing and refreshing to your entire face and sensatory organs such as eyes, ears, nose, mouth, tongue, and clearing your mind of mental congestion.

Make sure you keep your breathing natural and comfortable, and that you are letting go of your stress and awareness of the outside world. Unless you cut yourself loose, this will become no more than a physical exercise with limited benefit.

Six Sounds

Qi circulation is altered by certain soft sounds chanted together. They are:

Hur (Her), which impacts the Heart and eases thirst and dry mouth
Fu (Foo), which impacts the Spleen and eases indigestion and diarrhea
Hui (Hoo-ee), which impacts the Lung and eases Cold cough
Shi (She), which impacts the Triple Burner and eases chest pain
Shiu (She-oo), which impacts the Liver and eases liver pain and inflammation
Chuei (Chew-ee), which impacts the Kidney and eases pain in the waist region and joints

The six sounds should be done in one smooth, barely audible chant during one exhale.

QI GONG FULL-CHANNEL MEDITATION

Qi Gong meditation is an extension of the physical exercises. Using focus and breathing techniques it also moves Qi, harmonizes the Shen, and strengthens the body's ability to fight disease. Any form of meditation is helpful in managing chronic disease and the anxiety that can accompany it. The following meditations are those used at Chicken Soup Chinese Medicine clinic.

Getting Started

Start slowly. Allow yourself to get into the proper frame of mind. If you expect too much too soon, you will disturb your mind/body/spirit.

Begin your meditation in comfortable surroundings. In the beginning you should try to eliminate as many distractions as possible: Choose a quiet, dimly lit room that is neither too warm nor too cold. Wear loose-fitting clothing.

Find a posture that works for you. You may sit on the floor, lie down, sit in a straight-backed chair, or stand.

Don't eat heavy foods or drink alcohol or caffeine before meditating.

Let go of disturbing thoughts. Meditation should help you set aside your worries for a while.

You may want to record the meditation on tape and play it back while you meditate so that you can follow the steps without having to worry about what you're supposed to do next. You may also have someone read it slowly and softly to you. When you are familiar with the routine, you can do it in silence.

The Routine

- Close your eyes. Close your mouth and place the tip of your tongue against the roof of your mouth. This connects the Yin and Yang channels and allows for Qi flow.
- With your eyes closed, bring your attention to the area around and below your navel where Qi is stored.
- Allow yourself to begin to breathe into the area. As you breathe into the abdomen, notice an ever-expanding warmth in the center of your abdomen.
- Notice the energy moving up into the area of your heart and opening up into your chest.
- Now notice as Qi moves to the area below your shoulder blades, and then on down the outside of your arms into your thumbs.
- When it gets to the tip of your thumbs, move your focus over to the index finger. Feel the Qi as it moves from your index fingers up the outside of your arms into the sides of your neck and then out onto your face beside your nose. Breathe in and out as it rests there for a couple of seconds.
- Then move it slowly to a spot under each eye. Feel it as it streams downward over your face and onto the front of your neck, heading over the front of your torso, down alongside the navel, and around the pelvic area until it comes to the outside of the thighs.
- From there it should move into an area just below the knees, and the Qi should feel particularly strong. From there it moves down the shins to the front of the feet and the tops of the toes.
- Spend time feeling the Qi in your toes. Begin along the inside of each big toe, along the arch, in front of the ankle bones, up along the inside of your legs and the front of your body, around the ribs, coming to rest along the outside of your ribs.
- Shift your attention to your heart. Feel how the Qi flows from there toward your armpit, down the inside of your arm. Bring it back up along the outside of the arms, across your collarbone, and up the back of your neck

to the front of your ears. Breathe slowly and peacefully for about thirty seconds.

- Begin again to find Qi as it moves from the inside corner of your eyes, up across the top of your head, and down the back of your neck. At that point you will feel the Qi divide and follow two parallel courses along either side of the spine. These separate routes reunify at the buttocks, and Qi then moves down the back of the legs, around the anklebones, and into the little toes.
- Qi then moves up from the feet, up the inside of the leg, and around the navel.
- Move Qi up the torso to the front of the arms and then down the middle of the arms into the palms of the hands. Feel it travel into the fingers.
- Turn your attention to your fourth fingers and feel the flow move up over the top of the hands, up around the elbows, over the shoulders, up along the neck, and around the ears.
- From there it moves back and forth over the head and comes down the back of the neck, across the shoulders, down the side of the body, zigzagging again on the side of the body, and all the way down over the hips and the deepest point in the muscle of the body in the buttocks. Then it moves down the side of the legs, all the way down to the top of the toes, to the fourth toes.
- Focus your attention on the flow of Qi through the big toe—out across the top of the feet and up the middle of the legs until it goes by the genitals and up into the lungs.

This is the whole cycle of Qi through the channels. Rest easily, breathing slowly, and enjoying the infusion of energy and peace that you feel.

From Robin Roth, Health Educator

Meditation is recommended by many Western physicians as well as by practitioners of traditional Chinese medicine. Most brochures from hepatitis C organizations recommend meditating, and numerous people with hepatitis C swear by its benefits. Some of these benefits come from meditation's documented ability to reduce the negative effects of stress. Stress has been found to impair blood flow to the liver, which may trigger liver damage, affect inflammation of the liver, and release killer cells that contribute to liver cell death. However, when meditation (as well as hypnosis and acupuncture) stimulates the vagus nerve from the brain to the liver, the negative effects of stress on the liver seems to be lessened.[1]

In addition, meditation has been shown to be extremely beneficial in lowering blood pressure[2], helping to deal with chronic pain[3] and headaches[4]. Meditation and visualization are becoming more and more a part of supporting better sleep habits (insomnia)[5], treating anxiety[6] and depression. People who meditate have better long term health outcomes with such challenges as cancer[7], HIV/AIDS[8] and other life-threatening diseases. These studies and many others show the power of working with meditation, to improve health and to support people in dealing with chronic disease. There are many types of meditation that can be learned and practiced. Taoist meditation, mindfulness, Buddhist mantras, walking meditation, medical imagery, visualization, relaxation exercises, self-hypnosis— there is a different type of meditation to meet different people's inclinations and needs. A powerful but easy-to-use type of meditation called Applied Meditation developed by Margo Adair has been utilized in a CD developed especially for people with hepatitis C, *Self-Care for Hepatitis C ~ Applied Meditation for a Healthy Liver* (for more info, e-mail info@hepCmeditations.org.) Applied Meditation is an accessible approach that weaves together work with imagery, intuition and mindfulness. In the booklet accompanying the CD, Margo writes:

> Though we tend to view our bodies and minds as separate, they are not. They are both parts of our whole self and are in perpetual, intimate connection with each other. Applied Meditation can help you meet the multiple challenges that hepatitis C brings. Working with your mind's connection to your body will enable you to become an active participant in your healing journey. You will find it easier to manage stress, to be in tune with your body's needs, maintain healthy habits, and it will help your liver too.

Here's a short meditation that's a sample of the three longer meditations contained in the CD *Self-Care for Hepatitis C ~ Applied Meditation for a Healthy Liver* by Margo Adair and Robin Roth. See the Resource Section for more information about the CD and booklet. To sit back and listen to this meditation, go to www.hepCmeditation.org for a downloadable MP3 file.

How to Use This meditation.

- Create a comfortable place to meditate uninterrupted. Turn off your phone so you won't be disturbed.
- Sit or lie down with your back straight; feel free to adjust your position as necessary.
- As you read the meditation, relax, open your imagination, and give yourself permission to enjoy your experience.
- If tension arises, use your breath to release it.
- If you lose your focus of attention, or want to deepen your experience,

simply focus on the sensations of your breath, then return your attention to where you left off.

- Follow the suggestions as you read them, and also feel free to ignore them whenever you would like to spend more time focusing on something that has come up for you; then tune back in when you are ready. After you return to an outer focus of attention, take a moment to jot down or draw in a journal any insights, agreements, and challenges that emerged.

This meditation is designed to be used time and again. Your inner consciousness loves the familiar and repetitious. Hearing the same words over and over creates a sense of safety, allowing you to keep delving deeper. Repeat listening will create new neural pathways, keeping you aligned with your health goals and keep your healing path clear and accessible. You'll find that you work with the meditation in different ways at different times, working with some sections on one listening and other sections another time. Sometimes you'll actively engage with what you hear, other times you'll hear it in the background of your awareness, and occasionally you'll feel as though you slept through it. If this happens be assured that your unconscious mind hears the meditation and is working from a deeper level.

We recommend that you create a regular time in your routine to listen to a meditation.

SEVEN MINUTES TO LIVER HEALTH

Make yourself comfortable . . .

Focus on your breathing . . . Let your breath relax into its own natural rhythm . . . full and easy; breathing in and out. Let the rhythm of your breath caress you into a calm and relaxed state . . . breathing in calm . . . breathing out tension . . . breathing in and out . . . breathing in calm . . . breathing out tension. . . . Allow yourself to relax more and more with each breath. . . . Feel the sensations of breath rolling through. . . . Breath carries life – whenever you focus on your breath you'll find yourself feeling fully alive . . . centered . . . and relaxed.

Now bring to awareness what makes your heart sing . . . remember what you love . . . what brings joy . . . good moments in life . . . bring to awareness what makes your heart sing. . . . Choose a memory; remember your experience . . . remember the details. . . . Recreate the experience and let yourself enjoy it all over again . . . as though it were happening now. . . . Good feelings alive inside you now . . .

As you inhale imagine that your breath rolls right through this memory and gets charged with all this energy. . . . Breathe in and charge your breath with all this positive energy, sparkling energy. . . . Light . . .

Breathe out and send your breath to your liver. Imagine your liver breathing this wonderful healing energy. . . . Imagine that you send this good energy into your liver and your liver draws in healing. . . . Each breath fills your blood with healing energy. Imagine blood flowing easily through your liver, nourishing your liver; healing your liver. . . . As your liver exhales, it clears away everything that needs to be cleansed. . . . With each breath, your liver continues to heal. Imagine your liver immersed in healing energy. . . . Imagine your liver cleansing itself with each breath that rolls through . . .

However you imagine this, give your liver the particular energy it needs—you may want to offer it loving kindness, appreciation, strength, color, or song— whatever quality you like, imagine it, sense the quality . . . give your liver the particular healing quality that it needs to function well. Imagine your liver receiving this energy. . . . Imagine it functioning well . . . sense healing happening. Trust it.

Now envision the day to come. . . . Fill your day with positive energy. . . . Imagine moving through your day with *all* the energy you need. . . . Imagine moving though all your activities with ease. . . . Feeling calm . . . balanced . . . focused and clear. . . . Imagine this in detail. . . . Imagine pacing yourself to maintain good energy throughout the day and taking time to rest as you need to.

Imagine taking care of your liver as you move through your activities, paying attention to drinking lots of water and eating healthy food throughout the day . . . Detecting anything that makes your liver work harder and avoiding toxins . . . avoiding anything that's potentially harmful. Imagine all of this. . . . Imagine moving through your day, always keeping your healing in mind, and making the choices that promote your health . . . caring for yourself, caring for your liver. . . . Imagine being centered, calm, and clear throughout your day . . .

Breathe positive energy into these visions and charge them up, make them vibrate, sparkle, glow, sing with positive intention. Set the stage. Tell yourself about your day . . .

Feel free to take as much time as you like before you return to an outer focus of attention. Complete your inner work and come out of this meditation on your own. Take your time and open your eyes when you are ready. . . . When you *do* open your eyes, snap your fingers or tap your feet on the floor. Notice when you return to an outer focus you feel energized and calm; fully alert, clear, and relaxed. . . . And know that you heal with each breath you take.

Massage

Massage is a form of passive exercise that stimulates the Essential Substances and harmonious energy without an aerobic component. This can be very helpful to people who have advanced liver disease.

Torso Massage

If you can tolerate having someone touch your torso around your liver, this can be very soothing and helps disperse fluid. You may want to use oil infused with cinnamon to warm your belly if it is generally cold, or if you have loose stools and abdominal cramps due to Cold.

- Lie on a flat, firm surface. If needed, place a small pillow under your knees to take the strain off your lower back.
- Close your eyes halfway so there is less distraction.
- Inhale slowly and deeply.
- Glide the hands from the back of your neck to the front of your upper chest.
- Glide them over the chest with long, smooth strokes of the open palms. Repeat several times.
- Place the right palm on the stomach, above the navel. Place the left hand on top of the right.
- Rub the stomach gently in a clockwise motion. Repeat twenty to forty times.
- Using the first two fingers, massage a point about two inches above the center of each nipple. Circle your fingers over the left nipple, then the right nipple. This opens the lungs.
- Place the palms of the hands flat on each side of the upper torso. Move the Qi (from the point above the nipple) to the side and bottom of the lungs. Massage in a smooth, flat motion to the side of the torso, and then down to the diaphragm.
- Place the tips of fingers on the pectoral muscle by the crook of each arm. Massage in a circular motion, tracing a three-inch circle—from the top of the chest moving inward until both hands meet in the middle. Then travel down, continuing the circular motion to the lower rib cage, and move to the outside. Travel up along the sides of the torso. Repeat full cycle.

INTEGRATED TREATMENT PROGRAMS

13

The Basic Hepatitis C Help Program

Creating a program that combines Chinese and Western treatments has changed my life. I am confident that my diagnosis is always as precise as possible. I can track how my therapy is affecting my liver, and I am able to use a full arsenal of treatments to help my liver and my whole being—from mind to body to spirit—be as strong as possible. In a funny way it has simplified my life because now I don't waste time worrying about what I'm doing or not doing to take care of this disease, and I am not stressed and fatigued and off my feet.

—RICHARD J., 33, diagnosed in 1992, more than
fifteen years after infection

OVER THE long and often bumpy course of hepatitis C, it is in your best interest to keep yourself in peak health by watching what you eat, limiting the amount of negative stress in your life, exercising, and generally protecting your liver from unnecessary wear and tear. If you can adopt the basic principles of self-care outlined in this chapter, you will go a long way toward improving your quality of life and, in some instances, actually lessening or avoiding the unpleasant complications of hepatitis C.

FOUR SMART RULES TO LIVE BY

Follow these rules—particularly if you have a chronic disease such as hepatitis C.

1. Moderation in all things is not a bad idea and not as dull as it may sound. Check out chapter 9, Chinese Nutritional Therapy, for some great-tasting healthy recipes. And delve into the inner excitement that is Qi Gong, the exercise routine that provides energy and calmness together.
2. Details matter. It isn't enough to simply decrease stress, for example. If you try to relax using alcohol or drugs, you'll end up causing a lot of very destructive stress on your liver and other parts of your mind/body/spirit.

3. The healthy patient is the pushy patient. Insist on clear, understandable, and in-depth information about your tests, your health, and, in fact, about anything you think your health-care provider should be willing and able to do. This can include getting hard copy or e-mail copies of all your labs, as well as correspondence and reports from your doctors.
4. Take charge of your overall well-being, and you will be able to enjoy every day to the fullest.

To help you achieve these goals, we've put together a six-step program incorporating diet, nutritional supplements, exercise, meditation, self-acupressure, and moxibustion, and a regular schedule of interaction with your health-care practitioners.

STEP ONE: EVALUATING AND TESTING

Whenever you are feeling poorly for more than a few days, you should consider visiting your Western doctor for diagnosis and lab tests to find out exactly what is causing your discomfort. At the same time or subsequently, you may want to visit a Chinese medicine practitioner to see if the symptoms can be eased with Eastern therapies.

Make sure that all your health-care providers—your general practitioner, Chinese medicine practitioner, hepatologist, and whoever else you may see—know about each other and are aware of all the treatments you are receiving. You are in charge of your health and need to coordinate it so that you do not inadvertently run into trouble with treatments that should not be combined.

You may want to review the details of what to expect from a Western and Chinese diagnosis that are in chapter 5.

STEP TWO: KEEP A DAILY JOURNAL

For one to two weeks keep a daily journal and record the following:

- everything you eat and drink and the time you consumed it; see chapter 9 for a sample log
- any bodily symptoms and the time of day they appear
- your physical activities and how long you do them, whether they are exercise, work-related, or just happen to come up in the course of the day
- sleep patterns
- digestion and patterns of elimination and urination
- your emotions and when they arise
- your intake of drugs, prescription or recreational, alcohol, nicotine products,

and caffeine; note any reactions to their intake that you can identify at the time
- mental clarity or lack of clarity

At the end of a week or two take time to carefully read through the logs and cross-check symptoms (mental clarity, physical sensations, elimination habits, sleep patterns) with diet, medications, and nonprescribed drugs and alcohol. See what seems to correlate with symptoms. If you identify trouble spots, adjust your behavior and talk with your health-care providers. Take the journal to your health-care providers and discuss the correlations of symptoms and actions. You may also want to keep a Medications Watch List, much like in your daily journal, that tracks the medications you take: the time of day; dose; and any symptoms—positive and negative—you think may be related to the meds. See page 198 for complete instructions.

STEP THREE: CLEANSE YOUR SYSTEM

Follow the Five-Step Liver Support Diet Program for Chronic Hepatitis C Without Cirrhosis (see page 127) if your health permits. Then for general dietary health follow the guidelines on page 134 and do the following:

- Eat cooked foods mostly—they are digested more easily. Depending on your condition, you may want to eat some raw foods occasionally or daily. Do not eat foods directly out of the refrigerator.
- Generally drink warm or hot drinks. Drinking cold fluids puts out the digestive fires that are important to the assimilation of nutrients. Do not drink cold drinks directly out of the refrigerator.
- With Heat syndromes, avoid hot or warm foods such as ginger, garlic, turkey, chicken, mutton, shrimp, and heavy oils. Eat an increased amount of raw vegetables, juices, and fruits (no more than one-third of your diet).
- With excess Dampness, avoid fried foods and dairy products completely. Limit intake of tofu, and when you do eat it, cook it thoroughly, preferably with ginger and garlic. Eat carrots, barley, rice, corn, aduki beans, mustard greens, chicken, potatoes, alfalfa, and rye.
- Avoid alcohol.
- Limit intake of coffee, chocolate, and other highly caffeinated foods.
- Drink green tea. It has liver-protective and anticancer effects. However, with anxiety and depression, consumption should be limited if you are caffeine-sensitive.
- Take supplements to make sure you are getting the vitamins you need (see page 138 for more details).

- Take lactobacillus acidophilus; use the refrigerated powdered type as directed.
- Take a multivitamin, multimineral supplement; the powder capsule form is easiest to digest. Sometimes B complex vitamins cause nausea in people with hepatitis. Make sure the multivitamin supplies selenium and chromium.
- To get essential fatty acids, take one tablespoon a day of organic flaxseed oil, raw sesame oil, or evening primrose oil to promote prostaglandins. Helps decrease muscle aching and fibromyalgia symptoms. Should be refrigerated to avoid rancidity.
- Take low-dose carotenoids/lycopenes at 5,000 to 10,000 units per day. Do not take vitamin A. Vitamin E—400 to 1,200 IU per day—can help cell-mediated immune function, skin problems, and memory loss.
- Take vitamin C if you can tolerate it; some sources recommend up to 6 grams per day. Take until you experience gas or loose stools, then back off until you are comfortable.

Take additional supplements as recommended by a nutritionist or other qualified practitioner.

STEP FOUR: REDUCE STRESS WITH QI GONG EXERCISE AND MEDITATION

Practice the Buddha's Breath on page 179.

Use the Torso Massage on page 189 as a passive exercise.

The belly rub stimulates Qi and other Essential Substances without causing stress on the liver. It is particularly good for people with advanced liver disease. You can do this as a self-massage or have a partner do it for you.

Follow the Qi Gong Exercises in chapter 12 and, if interested, find a teacher locally to take classes.

STEP FIVE: USE ACUPRESSURE AND MOXIBUSTION TO STRENGTHEN YOUR CONSTITUTION AND EASE DISCOMFORT

Twice a week you can enjoy the great feeling of relaxation and repair that comes from self-acupressure and moxibustion.

Use self-acupressure to strengthen your constitution. See page 168 for instructions on self-acupressure and a diagram of points. Use the following: Stomach 36, Large Intestine 4, Liver 3, Lung 7, Kidney 3, and Spleen 6.

> **WARNING:**
>
> Do not use the point Large Intestine 4 if you are pregnant.

Ear acupressure is also an effective and simple way to help keep your Organ Systems in harmony. For complete instructions see page 169.

Self-moxibustion instructions are on page 172. Use these following points for general HCV treatment: Stomach 36; this is a major Qi point that tonifies and regulates Qi. It also harmonizes the stomach and the spleen, and is good for digestive disorders and fatigue.

Spleen 6 tonifies the Spleen, Kidney, and Liver Organ Systems. Ren 6 tonifies deficiency and Qi.

Acupuncture guidelines for practitioners are on page 175.

STEP SIX: CONSULT A TRAINED HERBALIST

Discuss with your practitioner the herbal formulas that we use at Chicken Soup Chinese Medicine and Quan Yin clinics to counter Toxic Heat and general syndromes associated with HCV symptoms. The herbal protocol includes immune formulas such as Cordyseng (¼ to ½ teaspoon, two to three times per day), Enhance, Tremella American Ginseng (12 to 20 tablets per day), or; liver formulas such as Hepatoplex One or Ecliptex (9 to 12 tablets per day), and Silymarin 80% standardized extract (600 to 800 milligrams per day), and possibly the anti-Toxic Heat, antiviral formulas Clear Heat (6 to 18 tablets per day). For more details see chapter 8, Chinese Herbal Therapy for Hepatitis C.

The Medications Watch List

If you are taking Western drugs for hepatitis C (interferon and ribavirin), herbal formulas or other medications, either prescription or over-the-counter, you should monitor yourself carefully for possible liver toxicity or other adverse reactions. Use this log as a model. You may make notes either daily or twice weekly.

Prescription drug(s) name _____

    Frequency _____

    Dr. _____

    Date started _____

    Side effects noted _____

    _____

Herbal formulas or single herbs _____

    Frequency _____

    Dr. _____

    Date started _____

    Side effects noted_____

    _____

Over-the-counter medications taken _____

    Date started _____

    Length of time taken _____

    Side effects noted _____

    _____

Recreational or street drugs and alcohol taken _____

    Quantity or frequency _____

    Side effects noted _____

    _____

14

Managing Digestive Dysfunction

INFECTION WITH THE HEPATITIS C virus can trigger flu-like symptoms, nausea, and gastrointestinal pain. These general digestive upsets can wax and wane over the years without signaling any significant progression of the disease or development of complications. If, as time passes, the liver's functions do become impaired by fibrosis, cirrhosis, or portal hypertension, then several specific digestive complications may set in. Insufficient bile in the small intestine may make it difficult to digest fats. A breakdown in the synthesis of proteins and vitamins may lead to a lack of important nutrients. Fluid metabolism disruptions may trigger diarrhea or constipation, gas, cramping, a general feeling of bloatedness, and a loss of appetite.

To soothe these symptoms and to help harmonize digestive functions, discuss the following treatment options with your health-care provider.

SELF-CARE TECHNIQUES

You can do a great deal to improve your gastrointestinal health if you take control of your diet, follow a regular, moderate exercise program, and reduce tension levels. Combine the following suggestions with the steps recommended in the Basic Hepatitis C Help Program on page 193.

Dietary Self-Assessment

As mentioned previously, we strongly recommend that you keep a daily journal that includes a log of your dietary habits for at least one week. You may be amazed to see exactly what you do or don't eat.

In your food log you should make note of everything you eat and drink, even little tastes that hardly seem to count, and the time you consumed them. You should also record your physical and emotional feelings during the day and when you noticed them. For example: "7:30 P.M.—Had a soda and a handful of chips. Joints feel achy. Very sleepy; grumpy."

Carefully track your food intake along with notes on your physical and emotional states, and you may see patterns emerge. You may be able to identify the foods that make you feel good and the ones that make you feel bad.

The goal is to determine the diet that gives you the most balanced energy, relieves gastrointestinal symptoms, and gives your liver a break so it doesn't have to process large quantities of fats or hard-to-digest proteins or toxins. Here is a sample worksheet:

DAILY FOOD AND DRINK LOG

Morning
Beverages (including type and amount)

1._____ Time _____

2._____ Time _____

3._____ Time _____

Foods (be specific, such as 2 pieces of white bread toast with butter)

1._____ Time _____

2._____ Time _____

3._____ Time _____

Afternoon
Beverages (such as water, soda, juice, and all alcoholic drinks)

1._____ Time _____

2._____ Time _____

3._____ Time _____

Foods (be specific, such as white bread sandwich of grilled Cheddar cheese with tomatoes)

1._____ Time _____

2._____ Time _____

3._____ Time _____

Evening
Beverages (such as water, soda, juice and all alcoholic drinks)

1._____ Time _____

2._____ Time _____

3._____ Time _____

Foods (be specific, such as fried or barbecued chicken with skin on or off, white
   meat or dark)

1._____ Time _____

2._____ Time _____

3._____ Time _____

Late Evening

Snacks (be specific—list beverages, types of ice cream or dessert, or midnight
   raids on the refrigerator)

1._____ Time _____

2._____ Time _____

3._____ Time _____

Physical and Emotional Feelings

You want to notice things like fatigue, energy levels, temper, mood, sweating,
   feeling chilly, nausea, gas, nervousness, anxiety, depression, hyperactivity,
   boredom, happiness, hunger, feeling stuffed, and lack of appetite. Make a note
   of the feeling and the time whenever you become aware of it.

1._____ Time _____

2._____ Time _____

3._____ Time _____

4._____ Time _____

5._____ Time _____

Evaluating the Results

At the end of a week, sit down with your log, and go through the following check-
list to evaluate the results.

Assess your meat-eating habits. Count up the number of times you ate red meat
during the week. If it is more than three, you should reduce your intake—even if
you don't have cirrhosis or encephalopathy.

Estimate how many ounces of animal protein you ate in a week. USDA guidelines recommend no more than two to three servings of 2 to 3 ounces a day—and
that's for people with healthy livers. One large hamburger has about 6 ounces; a
half a chicken breast can be up to 8 ounces.

In Chinese medicine, meat is used as flavoring and an adjunct to grains
and vegetables. It is a valuable part of a balanced diet, but only if eaten in
moderation. In Western nutritional science, a lot of attention has been paid to
the negative effects of a diet high in red meats; these include the possible

correlation of colon cancer and heart disease to excess fat, cholesterol, and digestive stress.

If you estimate that you eat more than 65 ounces of meat protein a week, you should cut back on meat and increase your intake of vegetables and grains. With that much meat in your diet, chances are your total fat and cholesterol intake is too high. Everyone should limit fat to 20 to 30 percent of daily calories; those with problems digesting fat or seriously elevated cholesterol levels or some complications of liver disease may need to be even more sparing. Those with encephalopathy should completely eliminate red meat from their diet but should then consume 80 to 100 grams of protein each day from soy and soy products, beans, legumes or chicken and fish. If protein consumption falls below 40 to 60 grams a day, you could be facing a dangerous loss of lean muscle mass. For protein consumption guidelines for anyone with hepatitis, see pages 135. Remember, before you make any dietary changes, discuss them with your health-care practitioner.

Count the number of servings of vegetables and fruits you've had in a week. A serving of vegetables equals approximately a half cup of cooked vegetables or one cup of leafy greens. A serving of fruit is approximately one piece of fruit, a half cup of chopped fruit or three-quarter cup of fruit juice. If you had fewer than thirty-five servings in a week, you need to increase your intake. The government's recommendations are two to three servings of fruit per day and three to five servings of vegetables.

Add up how much fried or fatty food you have eaten. Having even one portion of food a day that is high in fat—whole milk ice cream, candy, rich sauces or gravy, fried meats or sausage, French fries—is probably too much.

Make a note of how many meals were home-cooked and how many were eaten out. Of those eaten out, how many could be called fast food? It is much more difficult to eat low-fat food when you are eating out, and low-quality food with many additives, such as those served in fast-food restaurants, adds even more of a burden to your liver. If at all possible, try to increase the number of at-home meals you eat in a week.

Make note of how many meals you eat sitting at a table without the TV on, in a quiet and relaxed environment. In Chinese medicine you are not only what you eat but how you eat. Food should be consumed in a respectful manner, a calm environment and with appreciation of flavors, textures, smells, colors, tastes, and even sounds. This allows food to be absorbed into your body more harmoniously—and to repair disharmony more effectively—than food that you eat on the run, surrounded by chaos, and without taking the time to savor its gifts.

Look over the emotional and physical timetable you've recorded. Are you experiencing negative symptoms, such as fatigue, irritability, grumpiness, or gas, at the same time you eat certain foods? If you suspect that a certain food may be contributing to your discomfort, eliminate it from your diet for a week to ten days. Then reintroduce it and see if it causes the same symptom again. Sometimes a simple break will help ease the reaction. Sometimes you may have to reduce or eliminate your intake permanently.

Give Your Digestive System a Break

Try the Five-Step Liver Support Diet Program on page 127. It is designed to help those with hepatitis C reharmonize their whole system, but it is particularly effective for easing digestive complaints. It is also a useful way to make a transition to a new diet, free of fast foods and toxins and emphasizing whole grains, vegetables, and fresh fruits.

Learn to cook and enjoy congees, or rice soups. They can be easily prepared and provide support for the digestive system. The congees that help dispel digestive disharmonies are mung bean congee; pickled daikon congee, dry ginger congee and sweet rice congee. For complete instructions on preparing congee, see page 146.

Using Selected Supplements and Herbal Remedies

If you have liver disease, you should always consult all your healthcare providers before taking supplements or herbs to make sure they are suitable to your unique circumstances and that there is no conflict with other medications you are taking. For further discussion of supplements see chapter 9.

Possible choices include the following:

- Quiet Digestion: Chinese medicine formula relieves nausea and abdominal distension, increases the functioning of the Spleen Organ System, removes Dampness, and regulates the Stomach Organ System.
- Curing Pills (or Pills Curing, as they are sometimes labeled) are also Chinese medicine formulas recommended for nausea and distended stomach. They increase Spleen and Stomach Organ System functions, regulate the Middle Burner, and expel Cold Wind.
- Lactobacillus acidophilus: Eases dampness. Recommended dose is one quarter to one half teaspoon three times a day between meals.
- For abdominal pain, antigas medications such as simethicone are frequently helpful.

Exercise

If your digestive problems are a result of Stagnation or Dryness, moderate exercise, and/or Qi Gong can help move your bowels and dispel toxins. In addition, make sure you drink plenty of water before and after exercising so that you do not increase Dryness problems. Focus on Qi Gong exercises in chapter 12 to keep Essential Substances circulating and to dispel Stagnation.

Massage and Stress-Reduction Techniques

In addition to the meditations and breathing exercises in chapter 12, the following abdominal massage helps ease digestive distress by harmonizing the Liver, Spleen, Stomach, Gallbladder, Large Intestine, and Small Intestine Organ Systems.

- Lie on your back with a pillow under your knees. Place oil on your hands and rub together.
- Place your right hand on your stomach above your navel. Place your left hand on top of the right. (If you are left-handed, do the opposite.)
- Concentrate on the gentle inhaling and exhaling of your breath.
- Move your hands over your belly in a clockwise motion twenty to forty times, until you feel warmth under your hands.
- Separate your hands so that each palm covers one side of your lower rib cage, above your belly button. Fingers should point toward each other. Massage down over your lower abdomen into your groin area. Repeat five times.
- Rub your hip bones with your open palms, following the contour to the top of your thigh. Repeat five times.
- Place your hands, one on top of the other, in the original position above your navel. Gently rub your belly with a circular motion. Remember to breathe in and out slowly and to concentrate on your breathing.
- Repeat these motions for up to fifteen minutes.

Self-Acupressure and Self-Moxibustion for Digestion-Related Syndromes and Symptoms

For instructions on how to give yourself acupressure, moxibustion, and massage therapy, see chapter 11. You can locate the following points on the drawings on pages 163 to 168.

Self-Acupressure Points for Easing Digestive Distress

For nausea: Pericardium 6, Ren 12, Spleen 4
For fatigue and weakness: Stomach 36, Spleen 4 and 6
For abdominal cramping and digestive upset: Stomach 25 and 37

Ear Self-Acupressure Points for Digestive Distress

(For more information on how to apply ear acupressure, see page 169.)

Spleen point: for treatment of diarrhea, chronic indigestion, abdominal distension

Stomach point: for low fever, abdominal distension, loss of appetite. For fatigue with digestive problems, do in combination with Ear-Spleen point.

Liver point: for Liver Qi Stagnation, irritability, gas, and fatigue that is relieved when you move around

Large Intestine point: for diarrhea and constipation

Self-Moxibustion Points for Easing Digestive Distress

WARNING:

Do not use self-moxibustion if you have diarrhea, fever, or bloody stools.

For Deficiency and Cold disharmonies: Stomach 36, Spleen 6, Ren 6 and 12, Stomach 25

For Xue and Qi Deficiency and Sinking Qi and diarrhea: Du 20

To tonify Qi: Stomach 36

For Dampness and digestive problems associated with Cold: Ren 12

For lack of appetite and weakness: Stomach 36 and Spleen 6

For nausea: Ren 12 and 14, Spleen 6

WORKING WITH YOUR HEALTH-CARE PROVIDERS

Digestive upset may occur as a result of the primary viral infection in reaction to Western medications or in response to raw herb formulas. Few stomach upsets are reported when herbs are taken in pills, tablets, or powders. Even if all you experience is minor nausea or a lack of appetite, such digestive problems can interfere with the quality of life and therefore deserve serious attention. Occasionally, digestive problems are the result of serious disease processes such as cirrhosis, portal hypertension, or ascites. That is why your health-care practitioner should always evaluate you if you have digestive complaints.

Your Chinese medicine practitioner may recommend the following:

- herbal formulas that target digestive problems; see chapter 8.
- acupuncture points for digestive upset that include these:

Nausea: P 6, Ren 12 and 14

Diarrhea: St 36, St 37, St 25 and Ren 6

Gallstones and gallbladder inflammation (cholecystitis): GB 24; gallbladder located 1 cun below GB 34. (This is a floating point called simply Gallbladder; it is only sensitive and activated in the presence of gallbladder disease.)

For Western medical treatment options see chapter 7, particularly the sections that deal with cirrhosis, portal hypertension, and ascites.

15

Dispelling Fatigue

FATIGUE IS ONE OF THE MOST PERSISTENT and troubling complaints associated with hepatitis C. Over the years or decades that hepatitis C remains a shadow illness, it may undermine your best efforts to maintain an optimal quality of life. Once hepatitis produces measurable complications such as cirrhosis, fighting fatigue may become a daily struggle. And frequently interferon therapy triggers overwhelming exhaustion, which is one reason that so many people find they cannot remain on the therapy for the full course of the medication.

Despite how common a problem it is, treating fatigue presents a challenge to both Western and Chinese doctors. If you experience persistent fatigue, you should visit a Western doctor for a blood test to determine if you have an undiagnosed coinfection or complication that is causing your weariness. At the same time you should explore the possibility that negative reactions to current medications and treatments might be causing the response.

In Western medicine, therapy for fatigue is available if the underlying disease trigger, such as elevated levels of ammonia in the blood, can be identified and there is a prescribed treatment plan. If the fatigue is free-floating and simply a by-product of viral infection, then the approach would be to use antiviral medications such as interferon to lower the viral load. Easing fatigue may be one of the long-term benefits—even if fatigue is a short-term negative side effect of the treatment.

In Chinese medicine there is a long tradition of treating fatigue associated with various syndromes and disharmonies. Before starting a program to combat fatigue you may want to be diagnosed by your practitioner; determining the nature of the fatigue is important before you begin treating it. One of the best ways to make a diagnosis is to ask the question, "Does exercise make my fatigue better or worse?" If exercise makes you more tired, then your fatigue is probably associated with a Deficiency syndrome. However, if you always feel more energized from exercise, then your fatigue is probably the result of a Stagnant Qi. When the precise syndrome is identified, your practitioner can coordinate your self-care and in-office treatments most effectively.

Once you have discussed your condition with your health-care provider, you may want to try the self-care techniques suggested below.

SELF-CARE FOR FATIGUE

The single most important tool for managing or overcoming fatigue, whether you rely on Western or Chinese medicine or some combination of both, is simply *rest*. It may seem a simple prescription, but many people try to steamroll over fatigue and end up making themselves more depleted and even more exhausted. This can lead to flare-ups of the flu-like symptoms associated with primary HCV infection or aggravate the symptoms of complications that are developing. Afternoon naps, a full eight hours of sleep a night, elimination of stimulants such as cigarettes and caffeine from the diet, and reduction of stress and tension are all important tools for managing fatigue effectively.

In addition to getting sufficient rest, Chinese medicine therapy suggests the following.

Adjusting Your Diet

As your liver becomes inflamed, it can have a difficult time synthesizing proteins and vitamins. You may develop intolerances to some foods and have trouble digesting others. Your intestinal motility may be reduced, leading to chronic constipation. Diarrhea can develop in reaction to viral flares. The liver may not be able to store glycogen as efficiently. Your whole intestinal system may become overtaxed and irritated, which may reduce the fuel you are extracting from the food you eat, and lead to lack of get-up-and-go and erratic blood sugar levels.

These symptoms can be eased by following the nutritional guidelines and principles outlined in chapter 9 and by following the guidelines below, which are designed specifically to ease fatigue.

- Eat five to six small meals a day instead of three large ones. This is less taxing on the system and may help keep blood sugar levels on an even keel.
- Rely on lower-fat meats and fish as well as plant-based proteins (whole grains, legumes, and beans) as much as possible. Do not overeat red meats or fatty processed meats.
- Drink sufficient water every day—at least 64 ounces. This is very important. Dehydration only exaggerates constipation and other intestinal problems.
- Do not eat many raw or cold foods. Try to stick with liquids that are room temperature and foods that are cooked. The body expends less energy digesting cooked foods.

Finding the Right Level of Exercise

Excess exercise can trigger a flare-up of symptoms for anyone who has hepatitis C. If you are already suffering from fatigue, it is particularly important that you don't overtax yourself. On the other hand, it is vital to oxygenate your system and maintain muscle tone if you are to stay as healthy as possible. The recommendations here are designed to help you restore energy whether you are so weary that you can't imagine exercising or you are so frustrated that you want to run the marathon.

- Take a deep breath. Even if you have severe fatigue, Qi Gong breathing and Qi stimulating movements can be done with minimal effort (you can even lie down to do them!) and still produce great results. Try Buddha's Breath on page 179.
- The cycle of three exercises—the Circle of Qi, Swing Low, Breathe Deeply and Qi Pumping on pages 179–180—will harmonize Qi and level out the highs and lows.
- As your strength returns, you can increase your routine. Add Zen Walking and more aerobic activities for ten minutes a day. *Always include the breathing exercises.* To decide if you are strong enough to add more vigorous exercise, ask yourself, "Could I walk comfortably at a steady pace for ten minutes? For twenty minutes?" If the answer is yes, then a daily ten or twenty-minute Qi Gong workout can provide the Qi nurturing and stimulation you need.

Keep the Fires Burning

Moxibustion one to three times a week is an effective tool for countering fatigue associated with Stagnant or Deficient Qi. Concentrate on Stomach 36, Spleen 6, Large Intestine 10 and Ren 4, 6, and 12. With a partner you can treat Urinary Bladder 13, 20, and 23 (you can't reach these points by yourself).

The Touch of Health

Acupressure

Acupressure on the channels and ear points is also very useful in easing fatigue and weakness. For instructions on how to perform self-acupressure, see page TK.

For fatigue and weakness: Stomach 36; Spleen 4 and 6

Ear Acupressure

In addition to the basic protocol outlined on page 168, follow these specific suggestions for a total of ten minutes once a day:

For fatigue relieved by activity and for Liver Qi Stagnation: Ear Liver, Ear Sympathetic, and Ear Lung

For fatigue with digestion problems: Ear Stomach and Ear Spleen
For fatigue related to negative side effects of medications: Ear Liver

Self-Massage

The Qi Gong torso massage (page 189) also provides a boost to sagging energy and moves Qi. Other self-massage points to rub ever so gently include Stomach 36, Kidney 3, Large Intestine 4, and Lung 7.

Acupuncture and Moxibustion

Treatment for severe fatigue and associated symptoms must be tailored to an individual diagnosis, but in each case an intensive routine for three to four weeks is recommended. Thereafter, monthly treatments are needed to maintain strength and vigor. Moxibustion will follow the individualized diagnosis that guides acupuncture. Suggested points for fatigue due to Deficiency are on page 176.

Herbal Therapy

All herbal preparations should be taken only under the supervision of a trained practitioner or medical doctor. Each syndrome associated with fatigue may require its own individualized herbal formula to complement the basic herbal protocol outlined on page 96.

One of the basic formulas, Enhance, is designed to target immune deficiency in conjunction with a viral disease and associated fatigue. Other traditional formulas such as Four Gentlemen tea may be prescribed to strengthen the body's energy. Six Gentlemen has additional herbs to strengthen digestion as well as increase energy. The main ingredients are astragalus and ginseng or codonopsis.

Marrow Plus is used particularly for fatigue associated with anemia-causing drugs such as ribavirin.

16

Immune-Strengthening Program

THE BODY'S *IMMUNE SYSTEM* is a somewhat mysterious and tremendously intricate world of offensive and defensive cells that work together to protect the body from disease—at least that's what they are designed to do. But in many instances, even though the immune system puts up a fight, its virus-killing soldiers are not able to kill off an invading bacteria or virus. In Chinese medicine terms, the Pernicious Influence overwhelms Protective and Normal Qi.

The thrust of most anti-HCV research, whether in China or the United States, is to find a way to help the immune system (Protective and Normal Qi) defeat the invading hepatitis C virus (a Pernicious Influence, to be sure). Many studies have confirmed that immune strength is strongly influenced by stress, mood, diet, and exercise. In this chapter are some self-care routines that you can use to bolster your immune system and strengthen its ability to fight off the results of infection. They may provide a useful complement to the therapy your practitioners prescribe.

SELF-CARE FOR IMMUNE STRENGTH

When your immune system is under constant attack, it needs help to build up its strength.

Eliminate the Negatives

The best thing you can do for your immune system is eliminate those stress factors that wear down your body's reserves and resiliency such as chronic tension or worry, which may cause irregular sleep patterns, an overcrowded schedule, unresolved conflicts with those close to you, irregular eating habits, smoking, recreational drugs, and reliance on stimulants such as caffeine and sugar to keep you going.

This is a tough list to break. We all tend to be particularly fond of those things that aren't good for us. However, the fact remains that resolving the underlying stresses and treating yourself better means reaping the rewards of more energy, a clearer outlook, and happier dealings with those around you. This overall feeling of being healthier puts you more squarely in control of your own health.

Breaking bad habits can be quite difficult, and you don't have to go it alone. There are terrific support groups for everything from smoking cessation to overcoming workaholism. Also consider consulting a nutritionist, trainer, yoga master, or psychologist to get the individual attention you may need to get your life back on track.

Increase Your Nutritional Fuel Supplies

Keep a daily log (see page 200) for a week. It can help you take an objective look at your diet and see if you have any nutritional deficiencies.

If you want to make changes in how you eat, aim to create a balance of food energetics. Remember, energetics are the power within food that cools or warms the metabolism and Organ Systems, moisturizes or dries the Organ Systems, and increases or decreases the flow of Qi, Jing, and Xue. Keeping energetics balanced is essential to maintaining harmony in Organ Qi and Protective Qi. For more information on energetics and nutrition in general see chapter 9.

Breakfast, the most important meal of the day, should contain a moderate amount of whole grains and protein. Lunch, the largest meal of the day, should contain a variety of grains, vegetables, fruits, and a small amount of animal or concentrated protein (three ounces). Dinner should be simple and free of stimulating, spicy foods and should include relatively little protein.

A balanced diet that strengthens the immune system and Protective Qi is not the result of simply following a nutritional formula. A balanced diet is the result of how you prepare your food and how you think about your food and what you eat. Balanced energetics are not simply the result of chemistry—they are also a result of spiritual forces.

Try the Five-Step Liver Support Diet Program on page 126 if you feel the need to cleanse your system and make a real break with your previous eating habits.

Use therapeutic foods that bolster Qi and Xue and strengthen your ability to fight disease. These include San Qi or Dang Gui Chicken or a congee made with American Ginseng, codonopsis, or red dates. (See the recipes in chapter 10.)

Engage in Moderate Exercise and Obtain Big Benefits

Moderate exercise is as important to a preventive health program as sound nutrition. *Excessive* amounts of exercise lower immune strength, trigger flare-ups in hepatitis symptoms, and worsen complications. The key to the success of moderate exercise is to find a reasonable and consistent pattern that works for you and then stick to it. Twenty to thirty minutes of walking a day, every day, is a whole lot better for your immune strength (not to mention mood and muscle tone) than running six miles once a week and then collapsing.

If you use Qi Gong breathing, exercise and meditation routines, either by themselves or in addition to other forms of exercise, you will reduce stress, harmonize your mind and spirit, increase your energy levels and strengthen your immune system.[1]

Target a minimum of 20 minutes of exercise a day, a maximum of one hour of exercise and or meditation, six days a week, is optimal. Remember, only you can really determine what is excessive and what is moderate exercise. Listen to your body and be attentive to what it tells you.

Use Self-Acupressure and Moxibustion for Immune Strength

Acupressure and moxibustion can strengthen Protective Qi. For instructions on applying acupressure see page 168; for how to use moxibustion see page 174. For the location of the points, see the drawings beginning on page 163.

Acupressure points to strengthen Protective Qi and the immune system: Stomach 36, Kidney 3, Ren 4 and 6.

WARNING:

Ren 6 should not be used during pregnancy.

Ear acupressure and massage: Give yourself a general ear massage for two to three minutes. Begin rubbing and pulling along the outer fold, particularly at the top front section, and then move into the inner cavities and end with the earlobe. Repeat on the other ear.

For overall rebalancing of Essential Substances and Organ Systems concentrate on the Ear Shen Men, Ear Lung, and Ear Spleen.

Moxibustion to tonify Essential Substances: one to seven times a week, Stomach 36. Once a week, Spleen 6, Ren 6 and 12, and Gallbladder 39.

Herbal Therapy

Herbal therapy is an essential step in strengthening Protective Qi. The modern approach is to use Fu Zheng herbs that are specifically selected to bolster the immune system. The basic herbal protocol for treating HCV contains several formulas that incorporate this principle, particularly Enhance, Tremella American Ginseng, or Cordyseng. These and all herbs are to be taken only under the supervision of a trained and/or licensed herbalist. Make sure to tell all your healthcare providers about the herbal formulas you take.

17

Relieving Depression and
Fuzzy Thinking

CHRONIC ILLNESS OFTEN TRIGGERS mental dysfunction such as depression, fuzzy thinking, memory loss, lethargy, and mood swings. With hepatitis C you may become depressed as a result of an underlying anxiety about being ill or from the anger and frustration caused by the limitations hepatitis can impose on life. Add to that the potential for changes in brain chemistry triggered by the viral infection itself, some of the specific complications of hepatitis C, and the side effects of antiviral medications, and you have a formula for emotional upset or turmoil.

It is important, however, not to simply accept feeling depressed or confused for weeks or days at a time. Have your Western doctor examine you to make sure you don't have encephalopathy or any other HCV-related complication that must be treated right away. In addition, you may want to consult a psychologist or psychiatrist for help in managing the stresses of living with a chronic disease. Your Chinese medicine practitioner also has many treatment choices to offer that are designed to resolve the disharmonies in the Shen and Organ Systems associated with your mental dysfunction.

There are two main Chinese medicine diagnoses associated with depression and general mental dysfunction: Shen disturbance and Lack of Shen.

Shen disturbance, when combined with Qi Stagnation, may lead to depression, forgetfulness, disorientation, insomnia, anxiety, digestive upset, chronic headaches, and irritability. It is associated with alcoholism and panic attacks. Even psychotic episodes can result. To restore balance to the Shen, various treatments are aimed at restoring the harmonious flow of Qi and Xue and balancing the Heart and Liver Organ Systems.

Lack of Shen produces different symptoms: The eyes are glassy and there is little engagement with the world—in short, you look as though the lights are on but no one's home.

After you have consulted your health-care providers, you may want to try some of the self-care techniques that Chinese medicine offers.

SELF-CARE FOR DEPRESSION AND FUZZY THINKING

Here is what you can do to create a self-care program.

Food for Thought

Dietary therapy can have a big impact on how your brain functions. Western medicine recommends that you treat the brain chemistry changes associated with high ammonia levels and encephalopathy, in part, by altering your protein consumption and eliminating red meat (see page 136). Mental fuzziness associated with glucose imbalances and the liver's loss of glycogen-storing abilities also calls for dietary adjustments. Alcohol and unsupervised drug consumption also have a profound negative impact on mental function. For help controlling your intake of these substances, see Addiction Management: Harm Reduction and Withdrawal, on page 221.

In Chinese medicine Shen disturbances that cause imbalances in Qi and Xue can be eased by making dietary adjustments.

To regulate Qi and create energy flow: your diet should contain basil, beets, black pepper, cabbage, chicken livers, coconut milk, garlic, ginger, kelp, leek, nori, peaches, and scallions.

To avoid Qi Stagnation: your diet should not contain alcohol, fatty foods, food additives, unnecessary medicines, or too many sweets.

To sedate excess liver: your diet should contain beef, chicken livers, celery, kelp, mussels, nori, and plums. It should not contain coffee, fried foods, excessively spicy foods, heavy red meat, sugar, and sweets.

To ease Xue Deficiency: your diet should contain oysters, sweet rice, liver, chicken soup, Dang Gui Chicken (see recipe on page 148). It should not contain raw fruit and vegetables, cold liquids, or ice.

One Step Forward

Qi Gong exercise and meditation soothes Shen and balances Qi and Xue. You should practice the breathing routines and exercises on pages 178 to 183 daily for twenty minutes.

At least three times a week, do the long Qi Gong Meditation on page 183.

Whenever you feel anxiety or tension try this five-minute meditation:

1. Lie down in a comfortable position with your eyes closed halfway.
2. Imagine a beautiful scene—a meadow, the mountains covered in snow, a tropical isle.
3. Let yourself smell the air, feel the sun on your face, hear the sounds of nature.

4. Using the deep, smooth Buddha's Breath (see page 179), breathe in the beauty of the imagined surroundings.
5. As you exhale, feel tension exit your body on your breath.
6. Wander through the scene in your mind, breathing in the lovely details and breathing out the bad feelings. Continue for five minutes.

You can add thirty minutes of aerobic activity—even walking—to your exercise routine if you do not become fatigued or experience a flare of hepatitis symptoms. Clinical studies show that exercise is one of the single most effective remedies for depression.

Clarify Your Mind with Acupressure Massage

Self-acupressure massage helps dispel Xue and Qi Stagnation and evens out your mood. When pressing on an acupoint, hold steady for a count of ten to thirty seconds, then move your finger around the point without lifting it from the skin for another count of ten. On the following points use a firm but not poking or rough touch: Liver 3, Pericardium 6, the Si Shen Cong—the four points on the crown of the head—and Yintang, between the eyebrows. (See illustrations beginning on page 163.)

Ear acupressure massage: Ear Shen Men, Brain, Heart, Sympathetic, and Liver points. See page 170 for location of points.

Acupuncture Guidelines

Practitioners often use the following points to improve brain function and ease mental anxiety or confusion: Du 20, Si Shen Cong (the four points on the crown of the head), Small Intestine 3, Urinary Bladder 62, Ear Brain, and Ear Sympathetic.

If the diagnosis is dementia associated with Wind and there are symptoms such as dizziness or numbness, then needle Large Intestine 2, Liver 3, and Gallbladder 20.

Consult a Trained Herbalist

WARNING:

All herbal preparations should be taken only under the supervision of a trained practitioner or medical doctor. Please refer to Appendix III: Liver-Toxic Medications and Herbs before taking any drug or herb. If you have any adverse reaction, discontinue use of the herb formula immediately.

An herbalist may prescribe the following formulas for Shen disturbances:

- Calm Spirit, a blend of Chinese and Western herbs and Western supplements;
- Aspiration, which nourishes the Brain and calms the Spirit;
- Ease Plus, or Bupleurum and Dragon Bone, to dispel Dampness and purge Heat. *Do not use if you are taking interferon;*
- Ginkgo biloba standardized extract, which has proved beneficial for memory loss in controlled studies.[1]

18

Easing Aches, Pains, Fibromyalgia, and Arthralgias

Hepatitis C frequently causes achiness, joint pain, and stiffness, probably as a result of the basic viral infection. It can also create arthritis-like symptoms if it triggers the formation of immune complexes called cryoglobulins, which can literally get stuck in and around joints. There is also some evidence that infection with HCV may increase the tendency to develop fibromyalgia, an often crippling disease of undetermined origin—most likely viral.

If you are suffering from such symptoms, you should have a blood test to determine if you have complications of hepatitis C that require specific or immediate treatment. You should then discuss with your health-care providers the best options available.

For general pains Western doctors may prescribe nonsteroidal anti-inflamatory drugs (NSAIDs) or even narcotics such as codeine. You want to beware of potential liver toxicity: Acetaminophen is safe in doses under two grams a day, but other over-the-counter and prescription pain relievers may cause side effects such as constipation, fatigue, nausea, dry mouth, and fuzzy thinking. If the side effects are troubling to you, investigate alternative medications. See below for various Chinese medicine treatments that are available.

SELF-CARE FOR ACHES, PAINS, AND FIBROMYALGIA

In addition to the Basic Hepatitis C Help Program outlined in chapter 13, you may want to try the following suggestions.

Stretching Out

With chronic pain, aerobic or weight-bearing exercise can overstimulate or aggravate sore joints and muscles. However, gentle Qi Gong exercises can dispel tension and help you relax.

It may also help to do mild stretching exercises, head rolls, hamstring stretches, or perhaps yoga, which gently massages each part of the body.

A mild full-body massage is also a terrific way to relax and extend tense muscles and joints. Be careful not to overstimulate or irritate the nerves and muscles. Avoid intense Shiatsu-style massage.

If your diagnosis indicates Dampness, Cold, and Deficiency, massage with warming and stimulating oils infused with cinnamon essential oil.

Meditation (see page 177) and the practice of mindfulness—being in the moment and quieting the mind—keep the mind from amplifying or fixating on pain.

Feel the Warmth

If you have not been diagnosed with a Heat disorder and do not have a skin rash or fever, you may find hot herbal compresses are very soothing. They come premade at health supply stores and herbal outlets, and you can also make them at home: Combine one cup of fresh rosemary, thyme, and mint. Wrap in a double-ply piece of cheesecloth and secure the ends. Immerse the cheesecloth package in a pot of boiling water. Remove from the water and wrap in thick towel. Place on your sore joints or muscles until the towel cools.

Herbal Formula Recommendations for Practitioners

All herbal preparations should be taken only under the supervision of a trained and licensed herbalist.

- Channel Flow is designed to work specifically on fibromyalgia and abdominal pain.
- Mobility 3 is for treating the lower body and joints.
- Mobility 2 is when inflammation is present.
- Ac-Q is for aching pain.
- Cir-Q warms and regulates Qi.
- Marrow Plus is for pain related to Deficient Qi and Xue.

Use Acupressure and Moxibustion

Using acupressure and moxibustion to ease pain can be done by your practitioner or at home. If you cannot reach these points yourself, ask a partner to lend a hand.

ACUPRESSURE POINTS:

- For upper back and shoulder problems: Pericardium 6 and Small Intestine 11
- For tendons, muscle pain, and tightness: Gallbladder 34
- For pain in the head and abdomen: Large Intestine 4, Pericardium 6
- To relieve Liver Qi Stagnation: Liver 3

EAR ACUPUNCTURE:

Stimulate the specific points that correspond to the areas of the body where there is pain. Also use Ear Sympathetic and Ear Shen Men. (See ear chart on page 170.)

Acupuncture Guide for Practitioners

- For pain related to Damp in the Channels: Spleen 6 and 9
- For pain related to Deficient Qi and Xue: Stomach 36, Spleen 6, Kidney 3, and Spleen 4
- For pain related to Stagnant Xue: Spleen 10, Large Intestine 11, and Spleen 6
- For pain related to Stagnant Cold: Ren 6 and Kidney 7
- For pain related to Heat or Damp Heat: Liver 2 and 5, and Large Intestine 11

Moxibustion can be applied on any area where there is pain without inflammation or redness. It is especially good over areas of pain as well as appropriate points.

Use it on the same points as listed in acupuncture above, unless the diagnosis is for neuropathy associated with Heat or Damp Heat. Then moxibustion is not recommended.

19

Addiction Management: Harm Reduction and Withdrawal

ADDICTION AND HCV ARE TWO TOUGH HEALTH ISSUES that people frequently have to confront simultaneously. Seventy to 80 percent of all new cases of HCV in this country arise as a result of substance use, especially IV drug use and shared drug paraphernalia such as straws and tissues.

Treatment for addiction is challenging: The success of detoxification depends on the physical and emotional abilities of an individual and the kind of support resources available. Programs for drug treatment are woefully scarce and often only temporary stopgaps. Poverty, mental illness, and discrimination all play a part in making it difficult for a person to overcome an addiction.

Some approaches are more effective than others, and many of those rely on the unique power of Chinese medicine, either as an adjunct to other programs or by itself. Heroin treatment programs have long relied on acupuncture—particularly ear acupuncture—to help heroin addicts through the initial stages of withdrawal. One of the wonders of the approach is that a person who is addicted will respond positively to acupuncture even if consciously resistant to detoxification. Treatments such as acupuncture are also effective in treating abuse of methamphetamines, cocaine, crack cocaine, tobacco, alcohol, and other chemical dependencies.

When complete withdrawal and detoxification is not a realistic goal, it is still important to use these therapies along with other behavior modification techniques to help minimize the risk of transmission of HCV between substance abusers and to encourage addicts to reduce their use of street drugs. Harm reduction is an important goal both for the health of the substance user and for society at large. At Quan Yin Healing Arts Center, director Carla Wilson advocates the following approach:

1. Working to prevent the initiation of drug injection, which avoids the infection risks associated with this behavior, and providing education and health outreach to help halt ongoing drug injection in order to eliminate future risks of HCV transmission. Substance abuse treatment can help the

person who injects drugs reduce the amount of drug use and perhaps eliminate it entirely.

2. Working to minimize the risk of transmission among injection drug users who continue to inject. This prevention strategy can reduce the chance that blood and blood-borne agents would be transferred among injection drug users. The harm reduction techniques include use of new sterile syringes and needles—not only for every injection but also for preparation of drug solutions—and the use of cookers, cotton, and water that have not been used by other injection drug users. The chance for transfer of blood should be minimal if these practices are followed. Changing the prescription and paraphernalia laws to make it easier for drug users to obtain, and possess syringes and supporting syringe exchange programs are important steps in achieving these safer injection practices.

3. Working to eliminate or reduce substance dependency in order to reduce the risk of coinfection with other genotypes of HCV or with other viruses including sexually transmitted diseases such as herpes and HIV.

4. Offering supportive treatments that ease withdrawal, restore nutritional support to the body, strengthen the immune system, and soothe the spirit. These treatments are outlined in the Eight-Step Program, below.

EIGHT-STEP PROGRAM

The goals of treatment are to calm the Shen; support the Spleen, Liver, and Kidney Organ Systems; and rebalance Qi and Xue. All the recommended dietary changes, massages, exercises, acupuncture therapy, herbal remedies, psychotherapies, and other treatments are designed to rebalance the body in these ways.

Following the program will help you move toward recovery. When recovery is not attainable, we urge you to recognize that any reduction in your habit is a positive step. You want to remove yourself from harm's way, but if that doesn't happen, you at least want to reduce the harm you inflict on yourself. As you go through this program, remember that you don't have to do everything at once. Take it one day at a time and work slowly to improve your strength and spirit. At each step, consult with your practitioner and your physician to make sure your liver disease is under control and you are not experiencing any other withdrawal-related complications.

Acute Withdrawal

The acute stage is when the physiological craving exists and physical withdrawal is in full bloom. You will experience severe headaches, difficulties with speech, irritability, anxiety, and possibly delirium tremens during severe alcohol withdrawal, and hallucinations during withdrawal from some other drugs, legal or illegal. Depending on the type of dependency, the reaction can last from a few days to a few months. In heroin addiction it can last up to two weeks, and methadone withdrawal may go on for up to a year. Withdrawal from methadone is long and slow. Methadone may stress the liver, complicating treatment for HCV.

Postwithdrawal Recovery

This is when the physical addiction is broken and the consequences of the physical damage become sharply felt. During this time and the long-term recovery stage, cravings, and the feelings of physical addiction can return, making it difficult to stick to the program.

Long-term Recovery

This is the time when all the physical, spiritual, and psychological disharmonies and disorders that the addiction itself created must be faced and treated. From a traditional Chinese medicine point of view, emotional consequences of severe liver imbalance require long-term treatment.

Chemical dependency also damages the Kidney Organ System, which is the seat of the Will. In all addictions the Will is compromised. Fear is also associated with the kidney. To strengthen the Will and quell fear, the kidney functions must be rebalanced.

The ability to address the underlying causes and results of substance abuse is what makes Chinese medicine so effective. Unlike other approaches that can do little more than mask the withdrawal symptoms, Chinese medicine creates the opportunity for people to strengthen and heal the mind/body/spirit.

Step One: Keep a Journal

For someone with HCV caught in the web of substance abuse, any use is too much as far as the health and harmony of your mind/body/spirit. But if you're ready to try a detox program, you know that already. If you're still using, keep track of your habits, how much you use the drug, how much money you spend on it, how it makes you feel, interactions and conflicts with those around you, and your physical and emotional responses.

For those of you who have gone through withdrawal already and are in recovery, keep track of your cravings, emotional and physical responses to withdrawal, and thoughts about staying off or going back to the drug. Try to stay aware of recurring problems that arise as your liver and body go through the process of detoxification. You may experience a dry drunk or become high even when you haven't ingested any substances. Being alert to these incidences can help you negotiate through them more easily. Also remember to make special note of positive improvements in your internal feelings and interactions with the outside world. Every day write out a list of the reasons that you want to successfully break dependency.

Step Two: Obtain a Western Medical Baseline

In order to develop a complete picture of the scope of your addiction and the damage done by HCV, go for a complete liver evaluation. Share your Western lab results with your Chinese practitioner and any other therapists you may use. Keep your Western doctor informed about the full range of treatments you are receiving.

Step Three: Follow Dietary Guidelines

Almost any addiction changes how people eat and affects the functioning of the digestive system. How many times have you quelled your hunger in the middle of the afternoon with a good, strong cup of coffee? Smoking is often used as a substitute for food, and alcoholics and street drug addicts are notoriously disinterested in eating. These changes in eating patterns often lead to sugar cravings and problems with low blood sugar (hypoglycemia). In addition, any chemical dependency strains the digestive system, making it sluggish and erratic. Think about what those legal drugs—coffee and cigarettes—can do to your bowels.

To help ease sugar craving and low blood sugar, rebuild the digestive system, and nurture the Qi:

- Try eating small meals frequently. Initially, you may do your best with six small meals a day that are high in protein and complex carbohydrates. Avoid fatty meats such as beef, sausages, ribs, and fried chicken; they make digestion more sluggish. Instead, eat broiled fish and chicken, whole grains, and beans, for protein that will sustain you throughout the day.
- Avoid all sugar, including fruits, for the initial period of withdrawal.
- Drink at least 32 ounces of water a day during withdrawal. Increase to 48 ounces in later stages. Check with your doctor if you are experiencing fluid retention, swelling, or ascites. You may not be able to take in so much liquid.
- Increase fiber intake to offset constipation associated with withdrawal.
  Once you are through the acute and short-term stages of detox, try the Five-Step Liver Support Diet Program, a cleansing diet (page 127) to set your system back in balance.

Detox also uncovers the full extent of immune system depletion that has happened as a result of the addiction. To bolster immune strength, take CoQ10

(Coenzyme Q10) and vitamin C to bowel tolerance—that is, until you have excess gas or loose stools. Then cut back until you are comfortable. Consult your practitioner for advice on taking selenium and zinc.

Step Four: Exercise/Meditation

During the acute stage it may be difficult to exercise, but if you can, it will release endorphins that can soothe withdrawal symptoms and help move toxins out of the body. Qi Stagnation, which is a common result of addiction, is also alleviated by aerobics. However, if you have cirrhosis or portal hypertension or other complications of HCV, you should not do aerobic or weight-bearing exercise. Qi Gong or yoga meditation and breathing exercises are both safe and helpful for repairing and reharmonizing your body. A blend of yoga, Qi Gong, and meditation, thirty to sixty minutes a day, will do a great deal to vanquish symptoms and help you to maintain resolve. Use the Qi Gong Full-Channel Meditation (page 183).

Step Five: Soaks and Saunas

Try a cool sauna, no more than 102 degrees Fahrenheit, for fifteen minutes. Scrub the skin with a soft bristle brush afterward, and shower in lukewarm water to remove toxins that have been sweated out through the skin.

Step Six: Acupuncture, Moxibustion, and Ear Acupressure

For more than two decades acupuncture has been used effectively in the United States to help cocaine, crack cocaine, heroin, and alcohol addicts break their addiction. It works, along with massage, to dispel agitation and ease the blocks that result from the toxins being released during withdrawal. It also overcomes the imbalances that come from poor nutrition and suppressed emotions. The Shen becomes calmed, the liver balanced, and the flow of Qi and Xue rebalanced.

The use of acupuncture for addiction therapy in the United States was pioneered at the Lincoln Detox Center in the Bronx, and that's where I first trained in acupuncture. The calming effects are astounding to witness: Imagine walking into a room with dozens of heroin or cocaine addicts going through detox, sitting quietly and calmly. Even those who come in agitated and talking compulsively join the others in quiet repose as soon as they have the five needles inserted in their ear points. When I saw that more than twenty years ago, I had no doubt about the power of acupuncture. Now, a new study from Yale University has found that among cocaine addicts attempting withdrawal, 50 percent of those using ear acupuncture were cocaine free, while only 24 percent of those using sham acupuncture, and less than 9 percent of those using relaxation techniques to help in their detox were drug free.

In the first stages of withdrawal from chemical dependency, treatments should be at least once a day, but sometimes twice a day is needed. Nicotine withdrawal requires daily treatment for three to five days, with follow-up once or twice a week during the first month. This is done in conjunction with self-massage of ear points or the use of small metal balls taped to the ear points that you can massage whenever the urge to smoke becomes overwhelming. (These are left on for three days.) Your practitioner will design a routine that is tailored for your individual needs.

You should do moxibustion during detoxification only on the advice of your practitioner. For those who have chronic Dampness as a result of their addiction, moxibustion on Stomach 36 and Ren 12 is beneficial. See pages 166 and 168 for diagrams showing these points. If you have any Heat symptoms—high fevers, a bright red face, or burning diarrhea—avoid moxibustion.

The general detoxification points used in practitioner-delivered ear acupressure are the Ear Shen Men, Ear Sympathetic, Ear Kidney, Ear Liver, and Ear Lung points. (See the diagram on page 170.) You may stimulate these for yourself to relieve withdrawal symptoms and you are encouraged to seek a licensed practitioner to give you acupuncture treatments as well.

Other points that you can use for self-acupressure include:

For alcohol detox: Ear Spleen and Ear Liver points, Ear Lower Lung and Ear Upper Lung

For tobacco: Ear Shen Men and Ear Lung—upper and lower

For crack detox: You may use acupressure on the acupuncture channel point DU 20. See page 166 for location of the point.

Step Seven: Self-Massage

Both self-massage and massage by a professional are extremely soothing during detoxification and extend the benefits that acupuncture provides. Not only does massage stimulate Qi and remove toxins from the body, but it makes you more tuned in to your body's sensations and related feelings. For self-massage routines, see chapter 12.

Step Eight: Herbal Therapy

All practitioners have their own favorite herbal formulas, but the following are examples of those I've found most effective: They are listed below, along with the companies that make them if they are proprietary.

Detox Tea. This is a special formula used at Lincoln Recovery Center in the Bronx. Michael Smith, founder and director, created the formula. It uses three parts chamomile and one part each of peppermint, yarrow, hops, skullcap, and catnip. The tea is taken nightly to help you sleep, and as frequently during the day as necessary to help ease symptoms of withdrawal. This tea is particularly effective in alcohol withdrawal.

Ease Plus from Health Concerns

Ardisia 16 from Seven Forests

Clear Air from Health Concerns

Schizandra Dreams from Health Concerns

Calm Spirit from Health Concerns

A LAST THOUGHT

Although Chinese medicine treatment and other approaches can do a great deal to help heal the problems associated with substance abuse and hepatitis C, without strong prevention programs to stop transmission, it is an endlessly frustrating battle. Needle exchange programs, harm-reduction practices, and a strong political and social will to help treat substance abuse are essential.

Are You Addicted or Dependent?

Before you decide you don't need this program, ask yourself: Am I addicted to anything? Many people say, "I can stop taking cocaine. I only do it for fun on the weekends." Or "I'm not an alcoholic. I only drink on weekends." They do not realize they are in fact chemically dependent. But if you have ever wondered if you have a problem, chances are you do. If you answer yes to any one of the following questions, you should seek professional help and support to unravel your dependency and restore your mind/body/spirit to balance.

Does your character change when you use the drug? Are you angrier? Friendlier? More at ease?

Is it very difficult or impossible to go for a few hours or days without the drug or alcohol without experiencing withdrawal symptoms?

Have you ever changed or rearranged your life in order to keep using the drug?

Have you ever put yourself in a dangerous situation to get the drug?

Have you lost money, a job, self-esteem, or a relationship because of your addiction?

Have you ever lost track of hours or a day while under the influence?

Have loved ones tried to get you to stop, but you've refused?

Although self-care and responsibility for your own sobriety are the cornerstones of recovery from addiction, no one needs to or should go it alone. Western medical therapy and monitoring, Chinese medicine, psychological support groups, twelve-step programs, individual psychotherapy, and healing techniques from many other traditions are essential for long-term success. Medical supervision of withdrawal is important to make sure you don't experience any complication.

20

The Optimum Interferon Protocol: Supporting Interferon/Ribavirin Treatment with Chinese Traditional Medicine

After I had my first liver biopsy, I was shocked to hear "Stage 4—cirrhosis." The doctors explained that while I needed treatment I had a low chance of success because of the length of time I had been infected (twenty-five years), my extremely high viral load and the fact that I had cirrhosis. So you can imagine how difficult it was to decide on what treatment to try—especially when side effects were potentially severe and the chance of success limited. But being told I was only ten years away from the liver transplant list got me motivated to do everything possible. I made healing my priority, and repeated that phrase to myself over and over as an affirmation.

I'm a health educator and was already using holistic health methods, so I researched, reached out, joined an HCV support group, learned Qi Gong and tai chi, improved my everyday health habits, and listened to an applied meditation tape in order to use the body/mind connection to endure treatment and promote success.

I also started receiving acupuncture every week on the day after my interferon injection. I felt like the acupuncture took the edge off that jittery, yucky interferon feeling and really smoothed me out. I did have some side effects from the interferon and from the ribavirin too, but I discovered that there was a traditional Chinese medicine treatment or herb that would ease the side effects of the Western treatments and boost their effectiveness. My doctor uses the word cured! My liver biopsy—two years after finishing treatment—showed marked improvement, no cirrhosis, no Stage 4. Mainly Stage 2. I'm still working on healing, getting acupuncture regularly, taking herbs daily, doing Qi Gong and tai chi and meditating. I feel better than I have in years. It wasn't easy, but it was so worth it.

—ROBIN ROTH, 59, diagnosed in 1996, successful treatment 2001–2002

THE POWER OF THE PROTOCOL

At Chicken Soup Chinese Medicine and Quan Yin Healing Arts Center in San Francisco, and in many clinics in the United States, Mexico, and Canada, Chinese medicine and integrative practitioners are using the Optimum Interferon Protocol to help people with hepatitis C who are receiving interferon/ribavirin therapy heal more effectively.

Who Is the Protocol Good for?

Western doctors suggest that the 20 percent of those infected with HCV who progress beyond Stage 1 are candidates for interferon, unless contraindicated by psychiatric disease or autoimmune problems. This includes people diagnosed with cirrhosis who do not have decompensated cirrhosis.

Also, people infected with genotype 2 or 3 of the hepatitis C virus may consider interferon/ribavirin-based therapy at any time or at any stage of liver disease, because the treatment effectively clears the virus 70 to 85 percent of the time. In people who are infected with genotype 1 of the HCV the therapy eradicated the virus only about 40 to 50 percent of the time.

In addition, people who have been diagnosed with Stage 0 or Stage 1 fibrosis of the liver and have significant symptoms associated with hepatitis C, such as cryoglobulinemia, an immune complex disease, or a coinfection with B or HIV, may receive immediate interferon/ribavirin therapy.

How Does Chinese Traditional Medicine Improve Treatment?

The goal of Chinese medicine is to help a person complete the full course of Western drug therapy by managing side effects and allowing the full dose of medication to be administered. This allows the best chance of clearing the virus. Clinical trials indicate that taking at least 80 percent of the interferon and ribavirin dose, at least 80 percent of the time, is crucial to achieving viral clearance at six months after stopping therapy.

Chinese medicine practitioners are able to help alleviate side effects and may be able to limit the suppression of bone marrow function associated with interferon/ribavirin treatment. Anecdotal reports from twenty-four patients who underwent Drs. Gish and Cohen's combined therapies, 90 percent have cleared HCV. Those reviewed had diverse genotypes, stages, ages, and lengths of infection.

Body acupuncture and auriculotherapy (ear acupuncture) are highly effective for treating side effects associated with interferon and ribavirin. They are also used when a person is trying simultaneously to reduce or eliminate drugs such as heroin, morphine, cocaine, alcohol, and nicotine.

What to Expect From Receiving the Optimum Interferon Protocol

Acupuncture and herbs—by regulating the blood, tonifying Qi, and clearing heat—help the liver function better and also have an anti-inflammatory, antifibrotic effect. This in turn decreases the progression of damage and alleviates symptoms of the condition. Chinese medicine protocols may also reverse damage already done to the liver. In short, the basic benefits include:

- an increased chance that you can endure and finish interferon/ribavirin treatment
- an increase in the incidence of clearing the virus
- a decrease in side effects; a decrease in the need for additional Western or allopathic medications
- improvement in liver function, including enhanced function during treatment
- decrease in inflammation and in liver enzymes; a slowing of the progression of damage and, therefore, of the stage of disease

Our experience is that the best results of the Optimum Interferon Protocol are seen in people who have consistently used Chinese traditional medicine therapy for six months to one to two years prior to embarking on interferon/ribavirin treatment. However, if Stage 2 to 3 fibrosis or cirrhosis (Stage 4) is present, interferon treatment should usually not be delayed. This needs to be discussed in detail with the treating Western physician.

When a qualified licensed acupuncturist and/or herbalist is familiar with both hepatitis C and the contraindications of herbs or herbal formulas in hepatitis C and during drug treatment, Chinese and Western herbal medicines may be used safely in conjunction with interferon/ribavirin therapy. The hepatitis C professional certification program for licensed acupuncturists, designed by Misha Cohen, trains practitioners in the use of the Optimum Interferon Protocol.

How To Put Together Your Treatment Team

Often a hepatologist or gastroenterologist may see a person being treated with interferon only once or twice, at beginning and end of treatment. Usually, the frontline contacts for managing treatment and care are the hepatologist's RN, the person's primary care doctor, and sometimes the alternative medicine practitioner. In Dr. Cohen's practice, she and her staff often are the main contacts during interferon/ribavirin treatment and work closely with the physician's staff—particularly the nurse treatment coordinator.

A nurse treatment coordinator is of utmost importance before and during treatment for communication of:

- what to expect with treatment;
- what potential problems accompany treatment procedures;
- how Chinese medicine therapy interfaces with Western treatment.

The treatment care nurse is often designated by the pharmaceutical company providing the drug treatment. Sometimes this service is offered by a treating physician's practice or an HMO's gastroenterology clinic.

Drug Company Treatment Services

The *Be In Charge®* *Program* is a free service for people with chronic hepatitis C and is sponsored by Schering Corporation. Schering offers support services during interferon treatment. They offer you your own Personal Nurse Counselor, who will answer your questions by telephone. You may also call on the Nurse Counseling service toll-free, twenty-four hours a day, seven days a week to speak with a nurse.

Pegassist® is a complimentary hepatitis C support program sponsored by Roche for health-care professionals and their patients. They have a twenty-four-hours-a-day, seven-days-a-week nurse hotline to answer questions about treatment, with translation available in 150 languages. One-on-one Nurse Care Coordinators give individualized support with regularly scheduled telephone calls throughout therapy as part of their services.

Both pharmaceutical companies' programs offer a broad range of services, education materials, and Web-based interactive media to help manage interferon-based treatment for hepatitis C. Both companies also offer patient assistance programs for those who are not covered by insurance or are underinsured and need help with payment for medications or help with insurance reimbursement.

Interferon/Ribavirin Side Effects—and What to Do

Most people experience several side effects from interferon and ribavirin treatment—although ribavirin is the more common trigger, especially during the first four to six weeks of treatment. Ribavirin is a highly toxic immune stimulator: it increases interferon's effects but can cause a severe decrease in red blood counts (anemia), and respiratory and other problems. Monitoring for severe side effects such as profound anemia is an important part of treatment follow-up and should be done as outlined in the Optimum Interferon Protocol. A complete blood count (CBC) should be checked every two to four weeks while on therapy. Successful completion of drug therapy is absolutely dependent upon management of symptoms due to side effects. Therefore it is important to report all symptoms that you may experience to all of your practitioners. They can then help you to maintain yourself on as close to full dose therapy for the full course of treatment.

Fortunately, often symptoms can be managed much of the time—although you may want to reduce your workload—or even not work during the initial phase of treatment.

SIDE EFFECT MANAGEMENT: WESTERN AND EASTERN MEDICINE

Fatigue

Get plenty of sleep, keep well hydrated, and eat well-balanced meals to maintain your weight, if possible. In addition:

- Acetaminophen (Tylenol): Less than 2 grams per day orally in divided doses can help combat fatigue, particularly premedicating prior to an interferon injection, if the fatigue is worse one to two days after an injection.
- Herbs, acupuncture, and moxibustion are all helpful in eliminating fatigue.

Headache

If you experience headaches:

- Nonsteroidal anti-inflammatory drugs (NSAIDs) such as aspirin and ibuprofen may be helpful, but generally should not be used in people with significant liver scarring or cirrhosis, who are at risk for gastrointestinal bleeding or renal failure associated with NSAIDs.
- For migraine, medications such as Imitrex may be helpful.
- Self-acupressure on LI4, GB20, and self or partnered head massage can relieve headaches (see acupuncture point charts on pages 163 and 164).

Fever

- Fever tends to be worse with the first few interferon injections. If you have one of more than 101° F for more than 24 to 48 hours—or *not* following an interferon injection—promptly a visit to the M.D. to check for an infection.
- Cooling baths with peppermint and other herbs can help with fevers.

Myalgias/Muscle Aching

Follow the steps for fatigue and headaches above and

- soak in a hot bath, or
- soak in herbs and/or Epsom salts to relieve pain.

Nausea

For nausea linked to ribavirin, take the ribavirin with food, or eat smaller, more frequent meals. Other helpful remedies include:

- ginger
- avoiding smells and foods that trigger nausea
- taking a prescribed antinausea medicine such as prochlorperazine (Compazine)
- receiving acupressure on P6 (see points chart on page 165)

Anorexia

If you simply have no appetite or cannot eat regular meals, try:

- eating smaller, more frequent meals
- eating nutrient bars and protein for extra calories and protein in a day
- Moxibustion on St36 and Ren 12 can stimulate appetite (see points charts on pages 166 and 168).

Diarrhea

If your stomach and intestines become upset, try:

- Curing Pills or Quiet Digestion (Chinese herbal formulas), along with other herbs prescribed by a qualified herbalist specific to the Chinese diagnosis
- oral antidiarrheal agents drugs such as loperamide (Imodium) or diphenoxylate/atropine (Lomotil)
- avoiding or limiting caffeine-containing beverages and high-sugar soft drinks
- limiting lactose-containing foods
- eating boiled white rice, apples or applesauce, bananas, oatmeal, and bulking agents such as fiber supplements to help solidify stool

Insomnia

Lack of sleep makes healing that much harder. To sleep better, try:

- *not* sleeping during the day
- *not* reading or watching television in bed
- *not* drinking liquids before bedtime
- taking one gram (1,000 mg) of calcium/magnesium before sleep
- taking Calms Forte (homeopathic remedy)
- taking prescribed sleep aids such as diphenhydramine (Benadryl), Desyrel (Trazodone), or zolpidem (Ambien) as directed by a Western physician
- specific Chinese herbal medicines, according to the Chinese diagnostic pattern, prescribed by an herbalist

Irritability

Bad moods are common while on treatment. You and your near and dear should be aware that it may increase your temper and make you less understanding or patient. If you are aware that the medications may predispose you to temper flares, you can anticipate them and control them more effectively. In addition:

- make arrangements for job flexibility and limitation of stress at work
- use relaxation techniques such as deep breathing, Qi Gong; meditation, and self massage on P6 and H7 (see points charts on pages 164 and 165)
- share feelings with your friends and family
- join a support group

Depression

Depression develops in 20 to 35 percent of people treated with interferon and ribavirin. Health-care providers must screen for the development of severe depression or suicidal or other destructive thoughts. If you have a history of depression or other mental illness, seek ongoing treatment before interferon/ribavirin treatment is started.

- Selective serotonin reuptake inhibitors (SSRIs) may be prescribed by an M.D.
- Acupuncture has been shown to help alleviate depression.

Alopecia/Hair Loss

Approximately one third of people develop noticeable hair loss while on therapy. It tends to be gradual for the majority of people; however, the loss is subtle. To help protect your hair:

- Do not pull on hair or braid it, and avoid vigorous combing. Use a wide-tooth comb.
- Harsh hair products and chemicals should be avoided.
- Hair tends to grow back gradually to pretreatment quantity after interferon is stopped.

Skin Rash

Up to 25 percent of people on treatment develop a skin rash, usually from the ribavirin. It is a fine, red, petechial or reticular rash, and often occurs on the arms and trunk, although it may cover other areas. During the course of treatment it changes frequently, fluctuating between better and worse without much apparent reason. To manage it:

- Topical therapies, starting with moisturizing lotions and then low-dose steroid creams (for example, 1 percent hydrocortisone or triamcinolone), may be helpful in improving the rash and its associated itching.
- Wash with mild oatmeal soap to stop itching and improve hydration.
- An M.D. may prescribe oral medications such as diphenhydramine if topical therapies do not relieve symptoms. Chinese doctors also have herbal remedies that can be prescribed.
- In severe cases, dosage reduction or even discontinuation of ribavirin can be helpful, with reintroduction as symptoms improve. We generally do not recommend this, as it reduces treatment effectiveness.
- For skin rashes that develop at injection sites, changing sites is often helpful.

Anemia

The development of hemolytic anemia on ribavirin is dose-dependent. Dosage reduction of ribavirin manages symptomatic anemia, but the efficacy of treatment is dose-related, so your physician should only do this as a last resort.

Interferon can suppress bone marrow production of red blood cells. Anemia may result in more than 20 percent of those treated with a pegylated interferon and ribavirin at 1,000 to 1,200 milligrams a day. Anemia is one of the most clinically significant side effects. People with conditions that are made worse by anemia—such as coronary artery disease or chronic obstructive pulmonary disease—should be monitored very closely. People with HIV coinfection may be even more susceptible to developing treatment-related anemia due to treatment.

- Subcutaneous injections of recombinant erythropoietin can be used to treat anemia due to ribavirin.
- Marrow Plus (a marrow-strengthening herbal formula) is often used to help with the symptoms of anemia—however, there are no conclusive studies on its efficacy in conjunction with ribavirin treatment.

Neutropenia

Interferon suppresses bone marrow production of white blood cells, especially neutrophils, which leads to neutropenia in approximately 20 percent of people treated.

- Subcutaneous injections of filgastrim can be used to treat neutropenia due to interferon.
- Marrow Plus (a marrow-strengthening herbal formula) may help improve white blood counts—however, there are no conclusive studies on its efficacy in conjunction with interferon treatment.

Thrombocytopenia

Platelet counts also may drop during interferon and ribavirin therapy, possibly associated with interferon suppression of platelet production in the bone marrow. People with cirrhosis, who may begin treatment with low platelet counts due to portal hypertension, can be particularly affected.

- Manufacturer guidelines recommend reducing interferon dosage when the platelets fall below 80,000/μL, and stop interferon for platelets below 50,000/μL. However, individual M.D.s with much experience find that the platelet count can go much lower so this is up to each individual treatment plan
- Marrow Plus (a marrow-strengthening herbal formula) may help improve platelets—however, there are no conclusive studies on its efficacy in conjunction with interferon treatment.

Shortness of Breath (Dyspnea)

Shortness of breath is a common side effect of therapy, and it is often linked to the severity of anemia. Decreased hemoglobin and its oxygen-carrying capacity lead to shortness of breath upon exertion.

- A clinician should be consulted to evaluate shortness of breath in order to rule out serious cardiac, pulmonary, or other causes.
- Acupuncture may be used once serious causes that need to be treated by Western medicine are ruled out.

Chest Pain

A Western doctor should assess whether the chest pain is associated with heart conditions and what if any intervention is needed. Do not ignore symptoms.

- Acupuncture may be used to decrease pain.

Visual Changes

Visual changes are a fairly common side effect. The most commonly reported eye complications are "cotton wool spots" and retinal hemorrhages, but most interferon-related retinopathy is asymptomatic and reversible. A baseline eye exam should be done if you have any disease that is associated with retinal complications such as diabetes or hypertension.

- An ophthalmologist should evaluate anyone who develops visual changes while on interferon.

Thyroid Dysfunction

Interferon therapy can be associated with changes in thyroid function. Both hypothyroidism and hyperthyroidism may occur. Thyroid problems tend to occur more often in people with a history of thyroid dysfunction.

- Thyroid hormone replacement can be initiated if indicated.
- Acupuncture treatment may be used to improve thyroid function.

Other Side Effects

There are a number of other side effects associated with treatment that are not mentioned here—refer to the pharmaceutical companies' Web sites and ask your treating physician for more information. Also, www.hcvadvocate.org offers additional information on side effect management.

Optimum Interferon Protocol

Optimally, Chinese traditional medicine treatment should be started no less than twelve weeks prior to the first interferon injection. Dr. Cohen prefers to begin six months to one year prior to beginning interferon therapy. This will give the best results for completing interferon therapy effectively.

Twelve Weeks Before Starting Interferon Therapy

1. A licensed acupuncturist, Western physician, or other licensed provider should run baseline lab tests, including:

   - PCR (viral load) or other cellular testing such as TMA tests and bDNA tests;
   - complete blood count (CBC), including white blood count (WBC), hematocrit, hemoglobin, red blood count (RBC), differential (neutrophils/granulocytes, etc.), and platelets;
   - liver function tests, including albumin, and total bilirubin, including direct or indirect bilirubin;
   - liver inflammation tests such as ALT (alanine aminotransferase), AST (aspartate aminotransferase), GGT (gamma-glutamyltranspeptidase), etc.; and
   - international normalized ratio (INR) measured clotting time (previously known as prothrombin time).

2. At the same time, if the Chinese medicine program has not been begun prior to twelve weeks, the practitioner will begin the Chinese herbal treatment for hepatitis C:

   - hepatitis herbal pills (we use specific formulas);
   - immune formula (the herbalist's choice according to diagnosis);
   - marrow-strengthening herb formula; and
   - silymarin (standardized extract from milk thistle).

3. At this time, we also start the supplement plan:

   - Lactobacillus acidophilus: Use a refrigerated, powdered type (use dosage as directed on the bottle). This often helps many of the digestive problems that may be associated with hepatitis C. People who have taken many antibiotics or a high dose of antibiotics in the past may have very little naturally occurring lactobacillus acidophilus in the gut, which can lead to bowel disorders. Stool tests for pathogenic and beneficial bacteria are recommended in this case, to see if there is a deficiency in lactobacillus acidophilus. In this case, your doctor may recommend a higher dose than what is recommended on the bottle.

- Multivitamin, multimineral supplements in powder capsule form are best for digestion. B-complex vitamins may make some people with hepatitis nauseated. Make sure the vitamins provide an ample supply of selenium and chromium. It is best for people with hepatitis C that the formulas not include a lot of herbal substances, and herbs be provided separately, unless an HCV-knowledgeable practitioner has prescribed the specific formula. Ask your practitioner for help in determining your need for these formulas.

- Essential fatty acids (EFAs): Take one tablespoon per day of organic flax, raw sesame, or evening primrose oil to promote prostaglandins. Organic borage oil is effective for skin problems, such as itching and redness. Fatty acids help decrease muscle aching and fibromyalgia symptoms, and should be of the refrigerated type, in order to avoid rancidity.

- Low-dose carotenoids and lycopenes: Consume 5,000 to 10,000 units per day. (Do not take vitamin A.) Lycopenes are found in vegetables such as tomatoes, and have been studied extensively and been found to have anticarcinogenic effects. Many old-time vitamin manufacturers have recently added lycopenes to their formulas because of these recent studies.

- Vitamin E: 400 to 1,200 IU per day can help with cell-mediated immune function, skin problems, and memory loss. For people with severe bleeding disorders it is recommended to ask your physician before beginning Vitamin E intake.

- Vitamin C: If you can tolerate it, you may take up to six grams per day. Take to bowel tolerance (until you experience too much gas or loose stools), then reduce intake until comfortable. However, vitamin C should not be taken along with red meat, as it increases the uptake of iron, which may damage the liver further.

- Only a licensed nutritionist or a trained, qualified practitioner should recommend additional supplements. It is important that you consult your physician when adding a supplement program beyond the basic supplements recommended.

- Supplementation Strategy: For an additional supplement strategy, Dr. Lyn Patrick of the Hepatitis C Caring Ambassadors Program recommends what she considers an essential combination of 1,200 IU of vitamin E, 400 mcg selenium and 600 mg of alpha lipoic acid (ALA—from thioctic acid). She also recommends taking a combination of B vitamins along with this regime, as ALA can deplete the B-complex. For more information about her protocol please visit the Hepatitis C Caring Ambassadors online book *Choices,* at www.hepcchallenge.org.

Interferon Injections

It is a personal preference as to when to inject interferon. Some people choose to do it prior to the weekend in order to have time away from work if he or she feels ill from side effects. Others choose to inject in relationship to when they can receive acupuncture treatments. The timing of side effect symptoms post-injection varies a bit by several hours or a day. Therefore, each individual needs to work out the timing of injections with acupuncture treatments to relieve side effects along with other obligations. During the first four to six weeks of interferon treatments we often suggest that a person take a leave of absence or reduce their work load in order to adjust to the treatment schedule and to manage side effects in the best manner possible.

---

4. At twelve weeks prior to initiating interferon, we begin acupuncture therapy protocol treatment.

Two Weeks Before Starting Interferon Treatment

5. The Western or Chinese medicine provider should run all lab tests, including:

- PCR (viral load) or other cellular testing, such as TMA and bDNA tests;
- complete blood count (CBC), including white blood count (WBC), hematocrit, hemoglobin, red blood count (RBC), differential (neutrophils/granulocytes, etc.), and platelets;
- liver function tests, including albumin and total bilirubin, including direct or indirect bilirubin;
- liver inflammation tests: ALT, AST, GGT, etc.;
- INR; and
- TSH (Thyroid Stimulating Hormone).

6. At the same time, the Chinese medicine herbal practitioner individually modifies Chinese herbal treatments and supplements for each particular

client. This modification also includes the following very important suggestions (see chapter 8 regarding herbal interactions):

- discontinue silymarin;
- discontinue St. John's Wort and other related formulas; and
- discontinue any formulas containing chai hu (bupleurum).

7. Acupuncture treatments are increased to twice a week to prepare for any side effects during the beginning of interferon treatment.

During the First Week of Interferon Treatment

8. A CBC should be drawn, which can help determine the need for additional marrow-strengthening herbs or supplements. Sometimes discontinuation of certain herbs or supplements is necessary at this time. This is important in order to make a referral to the Western physician for medications when necessary.
9. Whether or not you have started the suggested acupuncture protocol 12 weeks before treatment, you receive an acupuncture treatment the same day or the day after the first interferon shot, depending on when your symptoms begin. You then should receive two acupuncture treatments per week for the first four-to-six weeks to relieve side effects most successfully.
10. Just prior to (minutes before) the first interferon injection, and usually prior to every injection, you should consider taking acetaminophen (Tylenol)—up to two grams per twenty-four hours—in order to prevent severe aching and reduce feverishness. Many clients swear by this as a way to prevent many side effects.
11. Drinking plenty of water infused with electrolytes such as Emergen-C also prevents many of the side effects associated directly with injection, including dehydration and skin and mucous membrane dryness.
12. Your qualified herbalist will increase or decrease herbs as necessary according to both Chinese traditional diagnosis and Western lab parameters.

During Weeks 2 to 4 of Interferon Therapy

13. In order to adjust herbs and supplements as well as refer to the physician for possible growth factor therapies such as erythropoietin (red blood cells) or neupogen (neutrophils/WBC), we recommend running a CBC.
14. In order to check for rapid viral response (RVR), we recommend running a PCR or other cellular tests on weeks two and four. Some HMOs and physicians do not include this in their protocols at the time of this publication.

It is a good idea to be proactive and ask for this. It can help the Western physician individualize the interferon therapy and help determine the timeframe and dosage of Western therapies.

15. At this point, the Chinese herbalist may adjust the marrow-strengthening formula according to labs as well as Chinese diagnosis.

During Weeks 5 to 24 (Genotypes 2 and 3) or Weeks 5 to 48 (Genotype 1)

16. We continue our Chinese traditional medicine treatment according to the individual's Chinese traditional diagnosis, as well as treating according to the lab parameters.

A current list of Hepatitis C Professional Certified practitioners (licensed acupuncturists and herbalists) can be found at www.docmisha.com. You can download the full list of certified practitioners in a PDF file and find a practitioner in your area. For those with no certified practitioner in your area, you can contact the NCCAOM for nationally certified herbalists and acupuncturists. You may also choose to have a phone consultation with an HCV certified practitioner. Please see the Resources section for additional information.

Epilogue (2006)

SIX YEARS LATER we have treated many people with HCV with a combination of Chinese and Western medicines. Alice Osiecki, now the coordinator of Living With Hepatitis C support group at Quan Yin Healing Arts Center in San Francisco, has this to say at the end of her successful hepatitis C treatment program.

I am living proof that the treatment program put together by Dr. Robert Gish and Misha Cohen works. I contracted hepatitis C in 1977 and was exhausted, plus I had a low-grade fever, gastrointestinal problems, brain fog, environmental sensitivity, insomnia, and depression. I went to a series of Western physicians and was told more than once that my problem was psychological. So I went to a psychiatrist to figure out if I was a hypochondriac. I also tried acupuncture. On my first visit the practitioner told me I had a liver/spleen problem. I began weekly acupuncture, took Ecliptex and Hepatoplex, and did medical Qi Gong and meditation. I went faithfully for the next five years and although it took some time, my symptoms went away and I was able to live a normal life. But I still hadn't been diagnosed with hepatitis C. Not until 1994 when I went to a new doctor, who was both an M.D. and trained in Chinese medicine, did I find out what was really making me sick. She didn't read my chart, wouldn't let me tell my history or various diagnoses. She closed her eyes and said, "Tell me your symptoms." When I was finished, she said, "I think you have hepatitis C." She referred me to a gastroenterologist who told me that I was not a candidate for treatment!

In 2004, I went to Dr. Gish's group, Physicians Foundation and finally received the Western medical care I needed. Searching for additional solutions, I went to a workshop at Quan Yin Healing Arts Center and heard Misha Cohen speak. I signed up for the Optimum Support Protocol that very day. Misha stressed the need for me to be proactive and be in charge of my health by putting together a holistic treatment program. I researched my disease, joined online hepatitis C forums, and faithfully attended the workshops and support group at Quan Yin Healing Arts

Center. I did acupuncture for eighteen months and meditated to Robin Roth's CD, *Self-Care for Hepatitis C.*

I finished my interferon treatment in 2006—and I had to contend with very few side effects, which I attribute to being on Misha's protocol. I was able to work all through treatment. It wasn't easy, but living with hepatitis C wasn't easy either. I recently found out that I cleared the virus!

We hope that the information in this book will help all those who have hepatitis C find the best path for their lifelong process of restoring balance and health to their mind/body/spirit.

Epilogue (2000)

THE BATTLE TO FIND an effective cure for hepatitis C continues. Until it is discovered, millions of people the world over must make difficult decisions about their treatment needs and choices, and fight against the often debilitating side effects of both the infection itself and available Western therapies.

As a society we need to offer help to those with hepatitis C. We should sharpen our focus on prevention; provide easier access to medical and psychological counseling and support groups; and fund cutting-edge research, including studies that explore the power of herbal medicines. The voices of the hepatitis C community are diverse, but they all echo one plea: Pay attention to this health threat. It is not someone else's problem. It touches us all.

Some of the most remarkable work is being done by people with hepatitis C who have come together to provide support to one another and lobby for change in the way our society is managing this epidemic. Alan Franciscus, founder and director of the San Francisco-based Hepatitis C Support Group and a patient advocate, is an example of the spirit and determination that characterize those with hepatitis C. He says:

> Having hepatitis C has changed my life entirely. My priorities have shifted. I take better care of myself, and I appreciate little things like being able to go for a walk in the park. And it inspired me to found the Hepatitis C Support Group.
>
> I started the group three years ago, about a year after I was diagnosed, because I personally discovered just how hard it is for people with hepatitis C to cope with the anxiety, the fatigue, and the confusion about treatment options. Plus, when you are too weary to think or to move, you can become incredibly isolated.
>
> Believe me, getting together with other people who have hepatitis C helps those who are newly diagnosed to get reliable information and to shake off the fear and stigma. The group is also helpful to people who are trying to make treatment decisions. Other people can share their firsthand experiences with you. And being in a support group helps those on drug treatment deal with very difficult side effects.

For me personally, the group has transformed me by bringing me into contact with incredible people and making me stretch myself. I do things I never thought I could do, like public speaking and putting together the newsletter. I think I'm most proud of the newsletter. It's the only one that's written by people with hepatitis C. And this is a group of very knowledgeable people—they often know more than their doctors about what's going on in research. With so much misinformation out there, it's important to have a source that is well researched and thoughtful.

But founding the group doesn't change everything in my life. I still have to contend with the same problems as anyone with hepatitis C. Treatment decisions are still tough to make. And there is a lot of stress and worry about the future.

Meditation and consensus interferon are my new approach to managing my hepatitis. This is my second try with interferon. The first time I took alpha interferon—what I call the demon juice—my liver enzymes went down to almost normal and my viral load was lower, although it was never undetectable. And a lot of symptoms I'd had for twenty years, like constant skin itching, went away. But I became terribly depressed. Nobody wanted to be around me. And there were other side effects like muscle aches, headaches, and constant nausea. I stuck with it for a year, though, taking three million units three times a week. At that time I also was getting acupuncture to ease some of the side effects and reduce my anxiety. I felt it was quite helpful.

A year and a half later, however, the fatigue became just unbearable again. I mean, I'm fifty and I have to be able to work to set aside money for retirement, but there was no way I could work full-time. So my doctor recommended that I take consensus interferon—the equivalent of five million units a day, every day for three months, and then cut back for the remainder of a year.

I started an antidepressant at the same time, something that everyone should consider when taking interferon, and I haven't had such a hard time. True, I sleep a lot—ten hours a day—and I nap in the afternoon, but I think it's worth it. Even if I don't get viral clearance, it does spare my liver while I'm taking it. The inflammation is reduced. And that may buy me enough time until scientists come up with a really effective treatment.

But I don't want to give the impression that a person with hepatitis C can just be a passive recipient of treatment. I believe that lifestyle changes are essential. You need to eat right, exercise, abstain totally from alcohol, and reduce stress. I meditate at least twice a day for around fifteen minutes. I use the techniques and ideas of Qi Gong, TM, and visualization. The first time I did it, I felt so good I got hooked.

I am an accountant by trade, but hepatitis C has changed how I define myself. Before I was diagnosed I was going through a career crisis of sorts. I went for an assessment of what other kinds of careers I might be suited for, and the counselor recommended teaching and health care. Well, here I am. Here we all are, together.

APPENDIX I:
Resources

EDUCATIONAL AND SUPPORT ORGANIZATIONS

AIDS Treatment Data Network (The Network)
The Network is a community-based, nonprofit organization that provides treatment access and advocacy, case management, supportive counseling, and information about AIDS/HIV and hepatitis.
611 Broadway, Suite 613, New York, NY 10012, phone 800-734-7104 x16 or 212-260-8868; fax 212-260-8869
www.atdn.org

Alternative Medical Forum (America Online)
This site has news, a resource directory, Internet chats, and places to ask questions about alternative therapies. Misha Cohen writes articles and participates in online chats through this forum.
AOL keyword AltMed or www.altmed.com

American Association for the Study of Liver Diseases (AASLD)
1729 King Street, Suite 200, Alexandria, VA 22314; phone 703-299-9766 fax 703-299-9622; e-mail aasld@aasld.org
www.asld.org

American Liver Foundation (ALF)
National voluntary nonprofit health agency dedicated to preventing, treating, and curing hepatitis and all liver diseases through research, education, and support groups. Misha Cohen and Robert Gish are on the Medical Advisory Committee of the Northern California Chapter.

75 Maiden Lane, Suite 603, New York, NY 10038; phone 1-800-GO LIVER (465-4837) or 212-668-1000; e-mail info@alf.org

Northern California Chapter: 870 Market Street, Suite 1048, San Francisco, CA 94102; phone 800-292-9099 or 415-248-1060; fax 415-248-1066; e-mail northernca@liverfoundation.org

www.liverfoundation.org/chapter/db/chapter/northernca, www.liverfoundation.org

ClinicalTrials.gov

The site is sponsored by the National Cancer Institute. It provides current information on many clinical trials.

www.clinicaltrials.gov

DocMisha.com

Misha Cohen's Web site contains information on hepatitis C, HIV, women's health, acupuncture, herbs and general Chinese medicine, and other traditional Chinese medicine therapies. It also features a question-and-answer forum where you can "Ask Doc Misha."

www.docmisha.com

Dr. Weil.com

This site has extensive information about integrated medicine.

www.drweil.com

Harm Reduction Coalition

The Harm Reduction Clinic fosters alternative models to conventional health and human services and drug treatment; challenges traditional client/provider relationships; and provides resources, educational materials, and support to health professionals and drug users in their communities to address drug-related harm.

East Coast Office: 22 West 27th Street, 5th Floor, New York, NY 10001; phone 212-213-6376; fax 212-213-6582; e-mail hrc@harmreduction.org

West Coast Office: 1440 Broadway, Suite 510, Oakland, CA 94612; phone 501-444-6969; fax 510-444-6977; e-mail hrcwest@harmreduction.org

www.harmreduction.org

HCV Advocate

Founded by activist Alan Franciscus, it offers a comprehensive site on all medical, social, and political aspects of HCV, plus information on alternative and Eastern therapies. The site publishes a newsletter that is a valuable resource with monthly updates on events, clinical research, and education; phone 415-587-8908; e-mail alanfranciscus@hcvadvocate.org

www.hcvadvocate.org

HealingPeople.com
Complete listing of acupuncturists and natural healers across the country. Has 500 Web pages covering all aspects of Chinese medicine for practitioners and consumers and many links to Chinese and alternative medicine Web sites. Also features excerpts from *The Chinese Way of Healing: Many Paths to Wholeness* and from *The HIV Wellness Sourcebook,* authored by Misha Cohen.
www.healingpeople.com

Health Central
Dr. Dean Edell's Web site contains sections on alternative and complementary therapies as well as the Hepatitis Conditions Center with numerous resources.
www.healthcentral.com

Health Concerns
Get information about the Health Concerns clinic, product information, newsletters, classes, conferences, books, and online shopping.
8001 Capwell Drive, Oakland, CA 94621; phone 800-233-9355; fax 510-639-9140; e-mail hconcerns@aol.com
www.healthconcerns.com

Healthology.com
Get answers directly from health professionals. Provides comprehensive overviews of common health conditions.
www.healthology.com/index.asp

Hep-C Alert
Provides advocacy, STD screening, support groups, and a national helpline: 877-HELP-4-HEP
660 NE 125 Street, North Miami, FL33161; phone 305-893-7992; fax 305-893-7998
www.hep-c-alert.org

Hep C Connection
Support groups and networking for people with hepatitis C. Also focuses on HIV and HCV coinfection.
190 East Ninth Avenue, Steward 320, Denver, CO 80203; phone 303-860-0800
www.hepc-connection.org

HepCMeditations
Information on using meditation and the body/mind connection to promote liver health. Guided meditations specifically for people with hepatitis C and other liver

challenges, downloadable, and for sale as a CD. Written by Margo Adair and Robin Roth. Self-care tips, resources, and personal stories.
www.hepcmeditations.org

HepNet (Hepatitis Information Network)
An excellent site if you are interested in learning more about the liver itself and its involvement in viral hepatitis.
www.hepnet.com

Hepatitis B Foundation
Good primary source of information for patients, their families and community. Includes information on treatments, research, and physicians.
700 East Butler Avenue, Doylestown, PA 18901-2697; phone 215-489-4900; e-mail info@hepb.org
www.hepb.org

Hepatitis C Action and Advocacy Coalition (HAAC)
Grassroots volunteer group committed to increasing prevention, treatment policies, and funding.
James Learned, 300 Eighth Avenue, #5A, Brooklyn, NY 99215; e-mail james_learned@ prodigy.net
Brian Klein, 530 Divisadero Street, Box 162, San Francisco, CA 94117; e-mail haac_sf@hotmail.com

Hepatitis C Advocate Network (Hep Can)
A volunteer organization representing persons living with hepatitis C.
www.hepcan.org

Hepatitis C Caring Ambassadors Program (HCCAP)
Dedicated to helping people with hepatitis C to equip themselves with all the facts and information about the illness and about the various treatment options available. The Hepatitis C Caring Ambassadors Brainstorming Team is: Terry Baker, Misha Cohen, O.M.D., L.Ac., Stewart Cooper, M.D., M.R.C.P., Randy Dietrich, Gregory T. Everson, M.D., Robert G. Gish, M.D., Randy Horwitz, M.D., Douglas LaBrecque, M.D., Peggy McCarthy, M.B.A., Lyn Patrick, N.D., Tina M. St. John, M.D., and Qing-Cai Zhang, L.Ac., M.D. (China)
P.O. Box 1748, Oregon City, OR 97045; phone 877-737-4372 or 503-632-9032; fax 503-632-9031
www.hepcchallenge.org
www.hepcchallenge.org/brainstorming.htm

National Hepatitis C Advocacy Council (NHCAC)
The council is a forum to discuss common goals in the effort to advance issues of importance to all people affected by hepatitis C.
www.hepcnetwork.org

Hepatitis C Support Project (HCSP)
HCSP is a nonprofit organization that addresses the lack of education, support, and services available for the HCV population. Bilingual materials are available.
P.O. Box 427037, San Francisco, CA 94142-7037; phone 415-587-8908; e-mail alanfranciscus@hcvadvocate.org
www.hcvadvocate.org/hcsp/hcsp.asp

Hepatitis Central
Information on herbs and answers to frequently asked questions, as well as an e-mail support list for hepatitis C and B.
www.hepatitis-central.com

Hepatitis Education Project
Provides educational materials and support groups for hepatitis patients and their families. Publishes a bimonthly newsletter.
4603 Aurora Avenue N., Seattle, WA 98103; phone 206-732-0311
www.scn.org/health/hepatitis

Hepatitis Foundation International
Supports research, educational programs, and materials for medical professionals, those with hepatitis, and the general public
504 Blick Drive, Silver Spring, MD 20904-2901; toll free 800-891-0707; 301-622-4200; fax: 301-622-4702
www.hepfi.org

Hepatitis Prevention, Education, Treatment, and Support Network of Hawaii (HEPTS)
HEPTS provides presentations and training opportunities for people with hepatitis and health-care professionals.
3254 Olu Street, Honolulu, HI 96816; e-mail kenakinaka@aol.com

HIV and Hepatitis.com
This is a great site that provides information for HIV and HCV and for coinfection, and articles on treatment options and studies. There is an extensive list of consulting editors who review all materials before posting.
www.hivandhepatitis.com

Institute for Traditional Medicine
Includes resources for practitioners and a list of clinics for treatment and information on herbal medicine.
2017 S.E. Hawthorne Blvd., Portland, OR 97214; phone 503-233-4907; fax 503-233-1017; e-mail itm@itmoline.org
www.itmonline.org

Integrative Medical Arts Group, Inc.
Provides resources and information for integrative health-care and educational and networking services to patients and medical professionals. IBIS, Interactive Body/Mind Information System, is an information database software on alternative medical therapies for medical professionals.
P.O. Box 671, Beaverton, OR 97075; phone 503-641-6060
www.healthwwweb.com

Lab Tests Online
This very informative site can help patients and caregivers better understand the many clinical lab tests that are part of diagnosis, monitoring, and treatment of an illness.
www.labtestsonline.org/understanding/index.html

Latino Organization for Liver Awareness (LOLA)
LOLA is a bilingual organization dedicated to raising awareness of liver disease through education, prevention, and treatment referral services.
P.O. Box 842, Throggs Neck Station, Bronx, NY 10465; phone 888-367-5652 or 718-892-8697; fax 718-918-0527
www.lola-national.org

National Department of Health and Human Services Center for Disease Control and Prevention (CDC)
1600 Clifton Road, Atlanta, GA 30333; e-mail cdcinfo@cdc.gov
Main www.cdc.gov
Hepatitis Information: www.cdc.gov/ncidod/diseases/hepatitis/index.htm
Prevention/Injection Drug Users: www.cdc.gov/ncidod/diseases/hepatitis/c/index.htm#idu

Misha Ruth Cohen Education Foundation (MRCEF)
MRCEF is a nonprofit organization dedicated to providing resources and education to medical professionals, patients, and the community. The foundation focuses on integrating western and eastern medicine in the treatment of a variety of complex health issues. MRCEF sponsors the Hepatitis C Professional Certification Programs as well as in-house training and internship programs for practitioners, students, and interested parties.

Phone/fax: 415-864-7234
www.hepatitisceducation.org, www.mishacoheneducation.org, www.tcmeducation.org

The National Center for Complementary and Alternative Medicine (NCCAM)
National Institutes of Health site for complementary medicine.
www.nccam.nih.gov

National Development and Research Institutes, Center for Drug Use and HIV Research
Funded by the National Institute on Drug Abuse.
www.cduhr.ndri.org

National Digestive Diseases Information Clearinghouse (NDDIC)
Offers patient education materials on hepatitis C. To obtain free copies, contact the
clearinghouse at NDDIC, 2 Information Way, Bethesda, MD 20892-3570; e-mail
nddic@info.niddk.nih.gov
www.niddk.nih.gov/health/digest/pubs/chrnhepc/chrnhepc.htm

National Institutes of Health (NIH)
The National Institutes of Health, a part of the U.S. Department of Health and
Human Services, is the primary Federal agency for conducting and supporting medical research.
9000 Rockville Pike, Bethesda, MD 20892
www.nih.gov

National Institute for Mental Health (NIMH)
NIMH provides national leadership dedicated to understanding, treating, and preventing mental illnesses through basic research on the brain and behavior, and
through clinical, epidemiological, and services research.
www.nimh.nih.gov

National Institute of Allergy and Infectious Diseases (NIAID)
NIAID research strives to understand, treat, and ultimately prevent the myriad in-
fectious, immunologic, and allergic diseases that threaten millions of human lives.
Contains a search feature to locate news, articles, and information.
Bldg. 31, Room 7A-50, 31 Center Drive MSC 2520, Bethesda, MD 20892-2520.
www.niaid.nih.gov

National Institutes of Health—National Library of Medicine (NLM)
News, general information, publications, information sources, and research programs. NLM collects, organizes, and makes available biomedical science information
to scientists, health professionals, and the public. The library's Web-based databases,

including MedlinePlus, PubMed, and PubMed Central, are used extensively around the world.

Main: www.nlm.nih.gov

Medline Plus: www.medlineplus.nih.gov

PubMed: www.pubmed.nih.gov

PubMed Central: www.pubmedcentral.nih.gov

National Institutes of Health Clinical Research Studies Protocol Database

Search the collection of research studies being conducted as the NIH Clinical Center.

www.clinicalstudies.inf.nih.gov

Medscape

Offers specialists, primary-care physicians, and other health professions an integrated multispecialty medical information and education tool. Provides clinicians and other health-care professionals with a source of clinical information.

www.medscape.com

National AIDS Treatment Advocacy Project (NATAP)

This is a scientifically oriented site with updated and comprehensive data on HIV and HCV.

www.natap.org

National Hepatitis C Advocacy Council

The National Hepatitis C Advocacy Council is an association of organizations that creates a unified voice, promotes ethical guidelines, and improves quality of services for people affected by hepatitis C.

P.O. Box 1748, Oregon City, OR 97045; phone 503-632-9032; fax 503-632-9031

www.hepcnetwork.org

Pharmacare

Provides comprehensive pharmaceutical care to clients living with challenging health conditions including HCV, HIV, AIDS, transplantation, and infertility.

695 George Washington Highway, Lincoln, RI 02865; phone 800-238-7828

www.stadtlander.com

San Francisco Department of Public Health: Disease Control Unit

101 Grove Street, Room 408, San Francisco, CA 94102; hepatitis prevention information line: 415-554-2844

www.dph.sf.ca.us

Substance Abuse and Mental Health Services Administration (SAMHSA)
U.S. Department of Health division for recovery for people with substance abuse
and mental illness also has sections on HCV/HIV coinfection.
www.samhsa.gov

USDA National Agriculture Library: Food and Nutrition
Provides links that feature the food pyramid, dietary guidelines, supplement information, the food safety research office, and more.
www.lincoln.nal.usda.gov/index.php?mode=subject&subject–al_nutrition&d_
subject=Food%20and%20Nutrition

VA National Hepatitis C Program
The Department of Veterans Affairs National Hepatitis C Program Web site, designed to be an informational and educational resource on viral hepatitis for health-
care providers inside and outside the VA system, veterans, and the general public.
www.hepatitis.va.gov

WebMD.com
Patient-driven Web site that features health and medical library, online chats, message boards, medical encyclopedia, self-care advisor, drug reference, "ask our experts," and more.
www.webmd.com

HEALING CENTERS

The following centers provide treatment for people with hepatitis C. You may contact them for an appointment, to arrange for a telephone consultation, or to request
literature.

Chicken Soup Chinese Medicine
Misha Cohen's private clinic. All treatments by appointment only. A limited number
of phone consultations are available.
Misha R. Cohen, O.M.D., L.Ac., Director; Corrina Rice, M.S.T.C.M., L.Ac., Assistant Director; Cindi Ignatovsky, M.T.C.M., L.Ac., Practitioner
San Francisco, CA 94103; e-mail chinmedsf@aol.com
www.docmisha.com

Fenway Community Health Center
Outpatient clinic with primary care services, mental health counseling, acupuncture,
chiropractic, massage, and acupuncture detox for alcohol and chemical addictions.

7 Haviland Street, Boston, MA 02115; toll free phone 888-242-0900 or 617-267-0900
www.fenwayhealth.org

Get Well Clinic
Offers herbal and nutritional counseling with master herbalists Fung Fung and Andrew
Gaeddert, as well as classes on herbs, Qi Gong, and Chinese massage therapy (Tui Na).
8001 Capwell Drive, #A, Oakland, CA 94621; phone 510-635-9778; e-mail
getwell@healthconcerns.com
www.healthconcerns.com/getwell.cfm

Robert G. Gish, M.D
California Pacific Medical Center, Liver Disease Management and Transplant Program
2340 Clay Street, #423, San Francisco, CA 94115; phone 415-600-1020; fax 415-
776-0292; e-mail gishr@sutterhealth.org
www.cpmc.org/advanced/liver

Immune Enhancement Program
Division of the Institute for Traditional Medicine. Offers treatment programs for
hepatitis C, HIV, and cancer using Chinese herbs and acupuncture.
2009 S.E. Hawthorne Blvd., Portland, OR 98214-3819; phone 503-233-2101
www.itmonline.org

Kang Wen Acupuncture Clinic
1111 Harvard Avenue, Seattle, WA 98122-4205; phone 206-322-6945

Lincoln Hospital Recovery Center
Provides acupuncture services for alcohol and substance abuse detox and recovery.
349 E. 140th Steward, Bronx, NY 10454; phone 718-993-3100

The Organization to Achieve Solutions in Substance Abuse (OASIS)
Comprehensive medical, mental health, support groups and vocational services for the
marginalized or addicted population with a focus on those infected with hepatitis C.
520 27th Street, Oakland, CA 94612; phone 800-282-1777; e-mail oasisclinic@
sbcglobal.net
www.oasisclinic.org

Lyn Patrick, NMD
Spiral Health Center; 129 E. 32nd, Durango, CO 81301; phone 970-385-9193; fax
970-385-9194; e-mail: lpatrick@frontier.net

Physician Foundation—Sutter Health Affiliate
California Pacific Medical Center, Liver Disease Management and Transplant Program
CPMC is a leader in hepatitis C treatment and research. The program offers complete hepatology evaluation, assessment and treatment for all liver diseases, including adult end-stage liver disease, and liver transplant to patients throughout California and Nevada. It performed its first liver transplant procedure in 1988, and has performed more than 1,000 transplants since.
Hepatologists: Robert Gish, M.D., Medical Director, Maurizio Bonacini, M.D., Natalie Bzowej M.D., Ph.D., Tami Daugherty, M.D.; Todd Frederick, M.D.; Stewart Cooper, M.D., M.R.C.P.; Ed Wakil, M.D.
2340 Clay Street, 2nd Floor, Room 224, San Francisco, CA 94115; phone 415-600-1020
www.cpmc.org/advanced/liver
www.cpmc.org/advanced/liver/patients/topics/hepc-default.html
Contact Sutter Health for a list of other affiliated clinics throughout California: www.sutterhealth.org/facilities

Portland Alternative Health Center
Division of Central City Community Health Services
Full-service Chinese and naturopath medicine for people with HIV infection and other health conditions related to drug and alcohol addiction.
David Eisen, L.Ac., M.S.W., O.M.D., Director
1201 S.W. Morrison Street, Portland, OR 97205-2219; phone 503-228-4533

Turning Point Acupuncture, Naomi Rabinowitz, M.D.
Private practice. Dr. Rabinowitz was affiliated with Lincoln Detox for several years and has many years of experience with HIV and Chinese medicine and fertility. Uses acupuncture and herb protocols.
1841 Broadway, Suite 509, New York, NY 10023; phone 212-489-5038
www.nycacupuncture.com

Quan Yin Healing Arts Center
Offers in-house and phone consultations. It offers the general public lecture series and classes, such as the Living with Hepatitis C Project, Hepatitis C Support Group, and Qi Gong. For practitioners there is the Quan Yin Professional HIV Certification Program and Quan Yin Professional Education Series.
455 Valencia Street, San Francisco, CA 94103-3416; phone 861-4964; fax 415-861-0579; e-mail qyhac@aol.com
www.qyhac.org

San Francisco City Clinic
Education and counseling, HIV testing, HIV services, hepatitis A and B vaccinations, women's health exam (Pap smear), pregnancy testing and urine testing for STDs. All services are private and free or low cost.
356 Seventh Street, San Francisco, CA 94103; phone 415-487-5500
www.dph.sf.ca.us/sfcityclinic

University of California, San Francisco—Liver Transplant Program
The liver transplant program is currently exploring the specific immune response of liver tissue, the use of transplantation with chemotherapy for liver cancer, regeneration of the liver, the study of cytokines (immune system regulatory agents) associated with liver transplant rejection, and prediction factors for recurring diseases.
400 Parnassus Avenue, 6th floor, San Francisco, CA 94112; e-mail lindag@itsa.ucsf.edu
www.gidiv.ucsf.edu/ltu/over.html

Zhang Clinic
Dr. Qing Cai Zhang's acupuncture clinic specializes in chronic viral diseases and autoimmune diseases.
420 Lexington Avenue, #631, New York, NY 10170-0632; phone 212-573-9584; fax 212-573-6639; e-mail yalezhang@cryticalsolutions.com
www.dr-zhang.com

Workshops, Classes, and Seminars

Doc Misha's Public Workshops and Professional Seminars
Dr. Misha Cohen, OMD, L.Ac. offers workshops for the general public and for health professionals for both the Eastern and Western medicine practitioners. She will also teach seminars on other topics upon request.
San Francisco, CA 94103; phone 415-864-7234; e-mail tcmpaths@aol.com
www.docmisha.com
Public workshops include the following:

> HIV/AIDS Wellness Programs
> Harmonious Cycles: Focus on Women's Health
> The Chinese Medicine Cabinet: Using Chinese Herbs for Optimum Health
> Hepatitis Help Programs including HCV and HIV/HCV coinfection

Professional seminars for Chinese medicine and other practitioners include these:

> Quan Yin Professional HIV Certification, a postgraduate professional training program for acupuncturists, Chinese medicine practitioners, and M.D.s trained in traditional Chinese medicine

Advanced HIV training seminars on digestive disorders, respiratory disorders, dermatological disorders, and women's disorders
Hepatitis C Professional Certification Course for Licensed Acupuncturists (other medical professionals may apply as exceptions)

HOW TO FIND A QUALIFIED LICENSED CHINESE MEDICINE PRACTITIONER

Contact the following organizations for referrals and certificate information.

Acupuncture and Oriental Medicine Alliance (AOMAlliance)
A professional membership organization of acupuncturists, Asian medicine providers, and acupuncture-related organizations.
P.O. Box 738, Gig Harbor, WA 98335; phone 253-238-8133; fax 866-698-8994; email info@aomalliance.org
www.aomalliance.org

American Association of Naturopathic Physicians (AANP)
The AANP provides referrals to naturopathic physicians and homeopathic practitioners.
4435 Wisconsin Avenue NW Suite 403, Washington, DC 20016; phone 866-538-2267 or 202-237-8150; fax 202-237-8152; e-mail: member.services@naturopathic.org
www.naturopathic.org

American Association of Oriental Medicine (AAOM)
Member-practitioner organization.
PO Box 162340, Sacramento, CA 95816; phone 866-455-7999; or 916-443-4770; fax 916-443-4766
www.aaom.org

American Medical Association: For Patients
Everything you wanted to know about the AMA and its physicians, including how to contact them. Also provides access to patient records and information.
www.ama-assn.org/ama/pub/category/3158.html

British Acupuncture Accreditation Board
63 Jeddo Road, London, W12 9HQ; telephone +44 (0) 2087-350400; fax +44 (0) 2087-350404; emailinfo@acupuncture.org.uk
www.acupuncture.org.uk/content/baab/baab.html

British Acupuncture Council
Register of practitioner members is published annually.
63 Jeddo Road, London, W12 9HQ; telephone +44 (0) 2087-350400; fax +44 (0) 2087-350404; e-mail:info@acupuncture.org.uk
www.acupuncture.org.uk

British Columbia Qualified Acupuncturists and Traditional Chinese Medicine Practitioners Association (QATCMA)
Professional Association promoting standardization, continuing education, and advocacy for the Chinese medicine professions.
#300—5900 No.3 Road, Vancity Tower, Richmond, BC V6X 3P7; phone 604-278-6220; fax: 604-278-1312; e-mail info@qatcma.org
www.qatcma.org

Chicken Soup Chinese Medicine Web Site
The Web site keeps an up-to-date listing of all medical personnel that have graduated from the Hepatitis C Professional Certification Course at: www.docmisha .com/applying/hepatitis_help/06download.html#certified
Referrals for Other Practitioners and Training:
www.docmisha.com/applying/practitioners_training/index.html

Greyston Foundation
21 Park Avenue, Yonkers, NY 10703; phone 914-376-3900; fax 914-376-1444; e-mail info@greyston.org

Healingpeople.com
Up-to-date and complete listing of acupuncturists and natural healers across the country.
www.healingpeople.com

National Acupuncture Detoxification Association (NADA)
Provides information on national and international drug and alcohol detoxification programs, and trains practitioners.
PO Box 1927, Vancouver, WA 98668-1927; phone 360-254-0186; fax 360-260-8620; e-mail nadaoffice@acudetox.com
www.acudetox.com

National Certification Commission for Acupuncture and Oriental Medicine (NCCAOM)
Can provide a list of nationally certified acupuncture, herb, and massage practitioners.

11 Canal Center Plaza, Suite 300, Alexandria, VA 2231; phone 703-548-9004; fax: 703-548-9079; e-mail info@nccaom.org
www.nccaom.org

WHERE TO STUDY CHINESE MEDICINE

The Accreditation Commission for Acupuncture and Oriental Medicine (ACAOM)
The main accrediting body for Chinese medicine schools in the United States. Maryland Trade Center #3, Greenway Center Drive, Ste. 820, Greenbelt, MD 20770; phone 301-313-0855; fax 301-313-0912
www.acoam.org

California Acupuncture Board
The official site of the State of California provides information on education, licensing, laws and professional associations. Contact for list of California approved schools. 444 N. 3rd Street, Suite 260, Sacramento, CA 95814; phone 916-445-3021; fax 916-445-3015; e-mail info acupuncture@dca.ca.gov
www.acupuncture.ca.gov

WHERE TO STUDY WESTERN HERBAL MEDICINE

California School of Herbal Studies
9309 Hwy. 116, Box 39, Forestville, CA 95436; phone 707-887-7457; e-mail cshs@cshs.com
www.cshs.com

WHERE TO BUY CHINESE HERBS

No one should use Chinese herbs without the recommendation and supervision of a trained herbalist. For the general public there are a limited number of herbs that may be ordered over the counter without a prescription. The following companies or centers provide quality products to practitioners and sometimes to consumers.

American Herbal Products Association
A more complete listing of suppliers of Chinese and Western herbs.
8484 Georgia Avenue, #370, Silver Spring, MD 20910; phone 301-588-1171; e-mail ahpa@ahpa.org
www.ahpa.org

Golden Flower Chinese Herbs
Golden Flower Chinese Herbs offers traditional and modern patent formulas manufactured with Spring Wind bulk herbs. They also carry products manufactured by Helio, KPC Herbs, Snow Lotus, and Spring Wind Bulk Herbs and Topical Products. 2724 Vassar Place NE, Albuquerque, NM 87107; phone 800-729-8509, 505-837-2040; fax 866-298-7541, 505-837-2052; email info@gfcherbs.com
www.gfcherbs.com

Health Concerns (for individuals and practitioners)
Manufactures a line of general formulas for the public and distributes other products such as echinacea and tiger balm. Also manufactures a line of high-quality Chinese herbal formulas that includes the hepatitis formulas designed by Misha Cohen. Maintains an herbal helpline for licensed practitioners. For the name of a licensed practitioner who uses the company's herbs, write or fax Health Concerns. Referrals are not given over the phone.
Andrew Gaeddert, President, Herbalist
8001 Capwell Drive, Oakland, CA 94621; phone 800-233-9355; fax 510-639-9140; e-mail hconcerns@aol.com
www.healthconcerns.com

Mayway Corporation (for individuals and practitioners)
One of the largest suppliers of Chinese herbal medicines in the United States. Produces a high-quality line, the Plum Flower brand.
1338 Mandela Parkway, Oakland, CA 94607; phone 800-2MAYWAY (262-9929) or 510-208-3113
www.mayway.com

Quan Yin Healing Arts Center (for individuals and practitioners)
People with a written prescription from their licensed practitioner may buy herbs from Quan Yin in person or by mail. Those without a prescription must have a consultation before receiving herbs.
455 Valencia Street, San Francisco, CA 94103; phone 861-4964; email qyhac.com
www.qyhac.org

WHERE TO BUY NUTRITIONAL SUPPLEMENTS

The following two companies are mentioned here because they supply supplements to Chicken Soup Chinese Medicine and Quan Yin. They may not sell to the general public but will recommend a practitioner in your area who carries these products. Many of the products are superior in quality and comparable to or lower in price than supplements available in health food and vitamin stores.

Karuna: Responsible Nutrition
Carries a wide variety of supplements and herbs for practitioner distribution only. I use this brand in my clinic for all the basic nutritional supplementation. I also use their Progesterone Plus, a natural progesterone cream.
42 Digital Drive, Ste. 7, Novato, CA 94949; phone 800-826-7225; fax 415-382-6147
www.karunahealth.com

Natren
A good source for acidophilus and pro-biotic products.
3105 Willow Lane, Westlake Village, CA 91361; phone 866-462-8736
www.natren.com

SELECTED BOOKS, CDS, AND PUBLICATIONS

Acupuncture: A Comprehensive Text
Chen Chiu Hseuh (Shanghai College of Traditional Medicine)
Translated and edited by John O'Connor and Dan Bensky (Eastland Press, 2002)
This is among the most authoritative textbooks and reference sources in its field. Since its translation into English in 1981, it has become a standard text used throughout the world.
www.eastlandpress.com

American Journal of Acupuncture
1840 41st Avenue #102, P.O. Box 610, Capitola, CA 95010; phone 831-475-1700; fax 831-475-1439
www.acupuncturejournal.com

Between Heaven and Earth: A Guide to Chinese Medicine
Harriet Beinfield, L.Ac., and Efrem Korngold, O.M.D., L.Ac. (Ballantine Books, 1991)
A very popular introduction to Chinese medicine and the Five Phases types.
www.amazon.com

Chinese Herbal Medicine, Formulas, and Strategies
Compiled and translated by Dan Bensky and Randall Barolet (Eastland Press, 1990)
The companion volume to *Chinese Herbal Medicine: Materia Medica*, this book of Chinese medicinal formulas in English serves as both a textbook for students and a major reference source for practitioners. Included are nearly 600 Chinese medicinal formulas arranged in 18 functional categories.
www.eastlandpress.com

Chinese Herbal Medicine: Materia Medica, 4th Edition
Compiled and translated by Dan Bensky, Steve Clavey, Erich Stoger, with Andrew Gamble (Eastland Press, 2006)
The primary study and reference text for the Chinese materia medica.
www.eastlandpress.com

Chinese Herbal Patent Medicines, Revised Edition
Jake Paul Fratkin (Shya Publications,)
This clinical desk reference book is a complete guide, providing a practical resource for acupuncturists, herbalists, naturopaths, as well as western doctors and veterinarians practicing natural medicine.
7764 Jade Court, Boulder, Colorado 80303; phone 303-554-0722; fax 303-554-0299; e-mail info@shyapublications.com
www.shyapublications.com

Chinese Herbs in the Western Clinic: A Guide to Prepared Herbal Formulas Indexed by Western Disorders & Supported by Case Studies
Andrew Gaeddert (North Atlantic Books, 1998)
This book is designed as a reference guide for practitioners who use prepared formulas (tablets and capsules) primarily, or as a follow-up or alternative to individually tailored decoctions.
www.northatlanticbooks.com

Chinese Medical Herbology and Pharmacology
John K. Chen, Tina T. Chen (Art of Medicine Press, 2003)
This is a modern pharmacology text on herbs and prescriptions.
www.jcm.co.uk

The Chinese Way to Healing: Many Paths to Wholeness
Misha R. Cohen, O.M.D., L.Ac., with Kalia Doner (iUniverse, 2006—Reprint of 1996 edition)
Offers comprehensive healing plans for a wide range of ailments including digestive problems, stress, anxiety, depression, addictions, gynecological problems, PMS, and menopause. These plans combine Chinese dietary guidelines with western medicine, plus various other eastern and western healing therapies.
2021 Pine Lake Road, Lincoln, NE 68512; phone 800-288-7800, 402-323-7800; fax 402-323-7824
www.iuniverse.com/bookstore/book_detail.asp?&isbn=0-595-39950-9

The Complete German Commission E Monographs: Therapeutic Guide to Herbal Medicines
German Institute for Drugs and Medical Products in the Bundesanzeiger, the German equivalent to the U.S. Federal Register. Translated and edited by Mark Blumenthal and Werner R. Busse (Lippincott Williams & Wilkins, 1st edition, 1998)
The text represents the most accurate information available on the safety and efficacy of herbs and phytomedicines. For physicians, pharmacists, and other health professionals.
www.amazon.com

CRC Handbook of Medicinal Herbs
James A. Duke (Wiley, 1985)
This handbook catalogs 365 species of herbs having medicinal or folk medicinal uses, presenting whatever useful information has been documented on their toxicity and utility in humans and animals.
www.amazon.com

Eating Well for Optimum Health: The Essential Guide to Food, Diet and Nutrition
Andrew Weil (Knopf, 2002)
www.randomhouse.com/knopf

The Encyclopedia of Natural Medicine, Revised 2nd Edition
Michael Murray and Joseph Pizzorno (Random House, 1998)
Naturopathic reference book for practitioners and consumers.
www.randomhouse.com

The Foundations of Chinese Medicine: A Comprehensive Text for Acupuncturists and Herbalists, Second Edition
Giovanni Maciocia (Churchill Livingstone, 2005)
This successful Chinese medicine textbook covers the theory of traditional Chinese medicine and acupuncture, and discusses in detail the use of acupuncture points and the principles of treatment.
www.intl.elsevierhealth.com/cl

The Green Pharmacy Herbal Handbook
James A. Duke, Ph.D. (St. Martin's Press, 2002)
www.amazon.com

The Green Pharmacy: The Ultimate Compendium of Natural Remedies from the World's Foremost Authority on Healing Herbs
James A. Duke, Ph.D. (St. Martin's Press, 1998)
www.amazon.com

Handbook of Chinese Herbal Formulas, Volumes I and II
Him-Che Yeung (Institute of Chinese Medicine, 1996)
These are compact handbooks that are perfect for clinic and classroom work.
www.ewbb.org

Handbook of Medicinal Herbs, Second Edition
James A. Duke (CRC Press, 2002)
This handbook catalogs 365 species of herbs having medicinal or folk medicinal
uses, presenting whatever useful information has been documented on their toxicity
and utility in humans and animals.
www.crcpress.com

Healing Digestive Disorders, Second Edition
Andrew Gaeddert (North Atlantic Books, 2004)
This book lists self-help strategies, treatment protocols and case studies for all major
digestive disorders. Designed for the professional as well as the layperson. It also
contains the story of how the author conquered Crohn's disease, a recommended
meal plan, workbook section, and acupuncture points.
www.northatlanticbooks.com

Healing Hepatitis C with Modern Chinese Medicine
Qing Cai Zhang, M.D. (Sino-Med Institute, 2000)
The book provides information on an herbal treatment program for hepatitis C.
www.amazon.com

Healing Immune Disorders: Natural Defense-Building Solutions
Andrew Gaeddert (North Atlantic Books, 2005)
Gaeddert offers hope for combating both simple and serious immune conditions using Chinese and Western herbs, supplements, diet, and lifestyle approaches.
www.northatlanticbooks.com

Hepatitis and Liver Disease: What You Need to Know, Revised Edition
Melissa Palmer, M.D. (Avery, 2004)
This book provides education about the disease and how to treat it with drugs, diet
and nutrition, alternative therapies, surgery and transplantation, the liver in pregnancy, as well as how to live with an imperfectly functioning liver.
www.amazon.com

Hepatitis C: A Personal Guide to Good Health
Beth Ann Petro Royball, M.A. (Ulysses Press, 2002)
This book details advances in therapeutic strategies and the search for a cure.

P.O. Box 3440, Berkeley, CA 94703; phone 800-377-2542; e-mail ulysses@ulyssespress
.com
www.ulyssespress.com

Hepatitis C
T. Jake Liang, Jay H. Hoofnagle, John I. Gallin, and Anthony S. Fauci (Academic
Press, 2000)
This is a volume in the Biomedical Research Reports.
www.amazon.com

Hepatitis C Choices, Fourth Edition
Hepatitis C Caring Ambassadors Program
The downloadable book is designed to provide a balanced view of the available treatment options and to help patients understand and make informed decisions on their
healthcare. Misha Cohen, O.M.D., L.Ac., and Robert Gish, M.D., are contributors.
www.hepcchallenge.org

Hepatitis C Forum
English version of a German site.
www.hepatitis-c.de/hepace.htm

The Hepatitis C Handbook
Matthew Dolan (North Atlantic Books, 1999)
www.northatlanticbooks.com

Hepatitis Magazine
Assists hepatitis patients and their families in taking control of their own health.
Misha Cohen is a contributing writer and writes periodic columns.
523 N. Sam Houston Parkway East, Ste. 300, Houston, TX 77060; phone 281-272-
2744 x132; fax 281-847-5440
www.hepatitismag.com

Hepatology
The official journal of the American Association for the Study of Liver Diseases.
www.aasld.org

The HIV Wellness Source-Book: Living Well with HIV/AIDS and Related Conditions
Misha R. Cohen, O.M.D., L.Ac. (Henry Holt, 1998)
Explains how to form individualized treatment programs and self-care plans that
combine Chinese medicine and Western science. The book presents a basic
comprehensive HIV+ regimen as well as targeted programs for treating digestive

disorders, respiratory problems, diarrhea, skin problems, fatigue, pain, anemia, depression, and more. Includes practitioner-assisted and self-care treatment programs for hepatitis.
www.amazon.com

Journal of the American College of Traditional Chinese Medicine
Although this journal is no longer being published, back issues and complete sets are still available from the college. They contain some excellent articles.
American College of Traditional Chinese Medicine, 455 Arkansas Street, San Francisco, CA 94107; phone 415-282-7600
www.actcm.org

Journal of Chinese Medicine
JCM Health Ltd., Unit 13, Langston Priory Mews, Station Road, Kingham, Oxfordshire OX7 6UP; phone +44 (0) 1608-659110; fax +44 (0) 1608-659529; e-mail info@jcm.co.uk
www.jcm.co.uk

Journal of Hepatology
Published on behalf of The American Association for the Study of Liver Diseases, *Hepatology* publishes original, peer-reviewed articles concerning all aspects of liver structure, function, and disease, such as immunology, chronic hepatitis, viral hepatitis, cirrhosis, genetic and metabolic liver diseases, and their complications, liver cancer, and drug metabolism.
www.hepatology.org

Living with Hepatitis C: A Survivor's Guide, Third Edition
Gregory T. Everson and Hedy Weinberg (Hatherleigh Press, 2002)
www.hatherleighpress.stores.yahoo.net

A Manual of Acupuncture
Peter Deadman, Kevin Baker and Mazin Al-Khafaji (Journal of Chinese Medicine Publications, 1998)
www.amazon.com

Natural Compounds in Cancer Therapy
John Boik (Oregon Medical Press, 2001)
A reference for those working in medicinal botanicals, offering a snapshot of the field of cancer treatment with nontoxic compounds in its infancy. This book is out of print but available for download.
www.ompress.com

Natural Therapy for Your Liver: Herbs & Other Natural Remedies for a Healthy Liver
Christopher Hobbs, L.Ac. (Botanica Press, 2002)
www.amazon.com

The Pharmacology of Chinese Herbs, Second Edition
Kee Chang Huang (CRC Press, 1998)
Herbal book by a pharmacologist trained primarily in Western traditions.
www.crcpress.com

The Practice of Chinese Medicine: The Treatment of Disease with Acupuncture and Chinese Herbs
Giovanni Maciocia (Churchill Livingstone, 1994)
A textbook for serious students of Chinese medicine.
www.intl.elsevierhealth.com/cl

Recipes for Self-Healing
Daverick Leggett with a preface written by Misha Cohen (Meridian Press, 1999)
Information on Chinese medicine nutrition, including wonderful recipes that use Western foods. In our opinion, this is the best book on Chinese traditional nutrition, with a great attitude.
www.redwingbooks.com

Self-Care for Hepatitis C: Applied Meditation for a Healthy Liver
Margo Adair and Robin Roth
A CD and thirty-five-page booklet that contains three guided meditations set to music that helps you tune in to what's happening in your body, promote good liver function, and facilitate a liver-healthy lifestyle. The booklet helps you get the most out of the CD, explaining how this accessible type of meditation works. Includes resources, personal stories and self-care tips. Online downloadable sample meditation, Seven Minutes for Liver Health.
Phone 415-287-0437; email info@hepcmeditations.org
www.hepcmeditations.org

The Treatment of Modern Western Diseases with Chinese Medicine: A Textbook & Clinical Manual
Bob Flaws and Philippe Sionneau (Blue Poppy Press, 2002)
www.bluepoppy.com

Warm Disease Theory
Wen BingXue, translated by Jian Min Wen and Garry Seifert (Paradigm, 2000)
First published in China in 1979 and translated into English for the first time, this is the standard text used by all institutes in China.
www.paradigm-pubs.com

The Web that Has No Weaver
Ted J. Kaptchuk (McGraw Hill, 2000)
The first widely popular book on Chinese medicine theory published in the United States. It is used as a textbook in Chinese medicine classes worldwide. Available from Amazon.
www.amazon.com

PUBLISHERS

Blue Poppy Press
This press and its founder, Bob Flaws, are well known in the world of Chinese medicine. The press sells books for practitioners and the general public on a wide range of Chinese medicine topics.
5441 Western Ave, #2, Boulder, CO 80301, phone 800-487-9296 or 303-447-8372; fax 303-245-8362; e-mail info@bluepoppy.com
www.bluepoppy.com

China Books and Periodicals
360 Swift Avenue, #48, South San Francisco, CA 94080; phone 800-818-2017 or 650-872-7076; fax 650-872-7808; e-mail info@chinabooks.com
www.chinabooks.com

Churchill Livingstone, a Division of Elsevier Books
Churchill Livingstone is a global publisher of health and medical books, journals, and CD-ROMs, including medical reference for health professionals and textbooks for lecturers and students.
Elsevier Journals Customer Service, 6277 Sea Harbor Drive, Orlando, FL 32887; phone 877-839-7126; fax 407-363-1354; email usjcs@elsevier.com
Elsevier Books Customer Services, Linacre House, Jordan Hill, Oxford OX2 8DP; phone +44 (0) 1865-474010; email eurobkinfo@elsevier.com
www.intl.elsevierhealth.com/cl

Eastland Press
Publishes textbooks for practitioners of Chinese medicine, osteopathy, and other forms of bodywork. Here you will find descriptions and reviews of each of our publications as well as information about the authors.
1240 Activity Drive, #D, Vista, CA 92081; phone 800-453-3278; fax 800-241-3329; e-mail orders@eastlandpress.com
www.eastlandpress.com

Eastwind Books & Arts
This independent bookstore stocks the nation's most comprehensive selection of both Chinese- and English-language books on traditional Chinese medicine and nutrition, t'ai chi, Qi Gong, Chinese divination arts, Feng Shui, and Chinese philosophy.
1435 Stockton Street, San Francisco, CA 94133; phone Chinese Dept. 415-772-5877, English Dept. 415-772-5899
www.eastwindbooks.com

Eastwind Books of Berkeley
2066 University Avenue, Berkeley, CA 94704; 94704; phone 510-548-2350; e-mail orders@ewbb.com
www.ewbb.com

North Atlantic Books
1435 Fourth St., Berkeley, CA 94710; phone 800-337-2665 or 510-559-8277; fax 510-559-8279; e-mail orders@northatlanticbooks.com
www.northatlanticbooks.com

Pacific View Press
P.O. Box 2657, Berkeley, CA 94702; phone 415-285-8538
www.pacificviewpress.com

Paradigm
Distributed by Redwing Book Co.
202 Bendix Drive, Taos, NM 87571; USA phone 800-873-3946; Canada phone 888-873-3947; worldwide phone 505-758-7758; fax 505-758-7768; e-mail custserv@redwingbooks.com
www.paradigm-pubs.com

Redwing Book Co.
202 Bendix Drive, Taos, NM 87571; USA phone 800-873-3946; Canada phone 888-873-3947; worldwide phone 505-758-7758; fax 505-758-7768; e-mail custserv@redwingbooks.com
www.redwingbooks.com

PHARMACEUTICAL COMPANY WEB SITES

Be in Charge Program (Schering Corporation)
Comprehensive patient education and support program that includes from maker of PEG-INTRON® (Peginterferon alfa-2b) and Rebetol® (Ribavirin). Includes a

personalized treatment diary, online support group as well as tips for managing side effects, energy levels, and exercise. Nursing support is available 24/7 at 888-473-2608. www.beincharge.com/bic/application

Hepatitis Neighborhood (CuraScript.com)
Excellent site that provides sections on treatment options, insurance, financial assistance, and a message board and support section.
www.hepatitisneighborhood.com

Infergen Aspire (Valeant)
Patient education and nursing support from the maker of Infergen® (Interferon alfacon-1). Nursing support is available 24/7 at 888-668-3393.
www.infergenaspire.com/wt/page/index8036

Pegassist (Roche)
Comprehensive patient education and support program, which includes information from the maker of Pegasys® (Peginterferon alfa-2a) and Copegasus® (Ribavirin, USB), a personalized treatment tracker, online support group as well as tips for managing side effects, energy levels, and exercise. Nursing support is available 24/7 at 877-757-6243.
www.pegassist.com

PreSCRIPT Pharmaceuticals Inc.
PreSCRIPT offers both brand name and generic medications from the manufacturers. They can provide a customized medical kit based an individual's needs.
www.prescript.net

APPENDIX II:
Herbal Formulas

BASIC PROTOCOL

Enhance (Health Concerns)
Ganoderma (Ling Zhi)
Isatis extract (Ban Lang Gen/Da Qing Ye)
Spantholobus extract (Ji Xue Teng)
Astragalus (Huang Qi)
Tremella (Bai Mu Er)
Andrographis (Chuan Xin Luan)
American Ginseng (Xi Yang Shen)
Hu Chang (Hu Chang)
Schizandra (Wu Wei Zi)
Ligustrum (Nu Zhen Zi)
White Atractylodes (Bai Zhu)
Cooked Rehmannia (Shu Di Huang)
Lonicera (Jin Yin Hua)
Salvia (Dan Shen)
Aquilaria (Chen Xiang)
Curcuma (Yu Jin)
Epimedium (Yin Yang Huo)
Viola (Zi Hua Di Ding)
Oldenlandia (Bai Hua She She Cao)
Citrus (Chen Pi)
Cistanches (Rou Cong Rong)
White Peony (Bai Shao)
Lycium Fruit (Gou Qi Zi)
Ho Shou Wu (He Shou Wu)
Laminaria (Kun Bu)
Eucommia (Du Zhong)
Tang-kuei (Dang Gui)
Cardamom (Sha Ren)
Licorice (Gan Cao)

Clear Heat (Health Concerns)
Isatis Extract (Ban Lan Gen and Da Qing Ye)
Oldenlandia (Bai Hua She She Cao)
Lonicera (Jin Yin Hua)
Prunella (Xia Ku Cao)
Andrographis (Chuan Xin Lian)
Laminaria (Kun Bu)
Viola (Zi Hua Di Ding)
Cordyceps (Dong Chong Xia Cao)
Licorice (Gan Cao)

Ecliptex (Health Concerns)
Eclipta Concentrate (Han Lian Cao)
Bupleurum (Chai Hu)
Milk Thistle (Sylibum)
Schizandra (Wu Wei Zi)
Curcuma (Yu Jin)
Tienchi (San Qi)
Salvia (Dan Shen)
Tang-kuei (Dang Gui)
Lycium Fruit (Gou Qi Zi)
Plantago Seed (Che Qian Zi)
Ligustrum (Nu Zhen Zi)
Licorice (Gan Cao)

Tremella American Ginseng (Health Concerns)
Tremella (Bai Mu Er)
American Ginseng (Xi Yang Shen)
Astragalus (Huang Qi)

Schizandra (Wu Wei Zi)
Raw Rehmannia (Sheng Di)
Lycium Fruit (Gou Qi Zi)
Lycium Bark (Di Gu Pi)
Isatis Extract (Ban Lan Gen/Da Qing Ye)
Lonicera (Jin Yin Hua)
Viola (Zi Hua Di Dong)
Ganoderma (Ling Zhi Cao)
Ophiopogon (Mai Men Dong)
Cuscuta (Tu Si Zi)
Dendrobium (Shi Ha)
Spantholobus (Ji Xue Teng)
Glehnia (Sha Shan)
Tang-kuei (Dang Gui)
Tortoise Shell (Gui Ban)
Epimedium (Yin Tang Huo)

Citrus (Chen Pi)
Curcuma (Yu Jin)
Licorice (Gan Cao)
Cardamom (Sha Ren)

GB-6
Ji Nei Jin (Ji Nei Jin)
Curcuma (Yu Jin)
Corydalis (Yan Hu Suo)
Taraxacum (Pu Gong Ying)
Melia (Chuan Lian Zi)
Salvia (Dan Shen)

Licorice 25 (Health Concerns)
Licorice root
Glycyrrhiza

HERBAL FORMULAS
FOR DAMP HEAT

Yin Chen Hao Tang
Yin Chen Hao (Artemesia capillaris)
Zhi Zi (Gardenia jasmoinides)
Da Huang (Rheum palmatum)

ADD THE FOLLOWING FOR
INTERMITTENT FEVER OR BITTER
MOUTH:
Chai Hu (Bupleurum chinense)
Huang Qin (Scutellaria baicalensis)

ADD FOR HYPOCHONDRIAC PAIN AND
FULL ABDOMEN:
Yu Jin (Curcuma longna)
Zhi Shi (Citrus aurantium)

ADD FOR NAUSEA, VOMITING, AND
INDIGESTION:
Zhu Ru (Phylostachys nigra/Bamboo
   shavings)
Shen Qu (Mass Fermenta
   Medicinalis)

Long Dan Xie Gan Tang
Long Dan Cao (Gentiana scabra)
Huang Qin (Scutellaria baicalensis)
Zhi Zi (Gardenia jasmoinides)
Ze Xie (Alismatis plantago)
Che Qian Zi (Plantago asiatica)
Mu Tong (Akebia trifoliata)
Sheng Di Huang (Rehmannia glutinosa,
   raw)
Dang Gui Wei (Angelica sinensis tail)
Chai Hu (Bupleurum chinense)
Gan Cao (Glycyrrhiza)

*Li Dan Pian (Qingdao Medicine Works,
tablets)*
Radix Scutellaria (Huang Qin)
Radix Saussurea (Mu Xiang)
Lysimachia Christinae (Jin Qian
   Cao)
Flos Lonicerae Japonicae (Jin Yin Hua)
Herba Artemesia Capillaris (Yin Chen)

Radix Bupleuri (Chai Hu)
Isatis tinctoria (Da Qing Ye)
Rhizoma Rhei (Da Huang)

Coptis Purge Fire (Health Concerns)
Coptis (Huang Lian)
Lophatherum (Dan Zhu Ye)
Bupleurum (Chai Hu)
Rehmannia (Sheng Di Huang)
Tang-kuei (Dang Gui)
Peony (Bai Shao)

Anemarrhena (Zhi Mu)
Akebia (Mu Tong)
Sophora (Ku Shen)
Scute (Huang Qin)
Phellodendron (Huang Bai)
Alisma (Ze Xie)
Plantago Seed (Che Quan Zi)
Gentiana (Long Dam Cao)
Forsythia (Lian Qao)
Gardenia (Zhi Zi)
Licorice (Gan Cao)

HERBAL FORMULAS
FOR QI AND XUE STAGNATION

Chai Hu Su Gan Tang
Chai Hu (Bupleurum chinense)
Bai Shao Yao (Paeonia lactiflora)
Zhi Ke (Citrus aurantium)
Chuan Xiong (Ligusticum wallichii)
Xiang Fu (Cyperus rotundus)
Gan Cao (Glycyrrhiza uralensis)

SOME SOURCES ADD:
Chen Pi (Citrus reticulata)

ADDITIONS FOR SEVERE ABDOMINAL
PAIN:
Yan Hu Suo (Corydalis yanhusuo)
Chuan Lian Zi (Melia toosendan)

Dan Zhi Xiao Yao San
Mu Dan Pi (Moutan radicis)
Zhi Zi (Gardenia jasminoides)
Chai Hu (Bupleurum chinense)
Dang Gui (Angelica sinensis)
Bai Shao (Paeonia lactiflora)
Bai Zhu (Atractylodes macrocephala)
Fu Ling (Poria cocos)

Bo He (Mentha)
Sheng Jiang (Zingiberis officinale) or
    Wei Jiang (stewed ginger)
Gan Cao (Glycyrrhiza) or Zhe Gan Cao
    (Glycyrrhiza, honey treated)

*Shu Gan Li Pi Tang (Spread the Liver
and Regulate the Spleen Decoction)*
Chai Hu (Bupleurum)
Bai Zhu (White Atractylodes)
Xiang Fu (Cyperus)
Dang Shen (Codonopsis)
Ze Xie (Alismatis)
He Shou Wu (Polygonum Multiflorum)
Dan Shen (Salvia)
San Qi (Notoginseng Powder)

Shu Gan Wan
Chai Hu (Bupleurum chinense)
Yan Hu Suo (Corydalis yanhusuo)
Bai Shao (Paeonia lactiflora)
Fu Ling (Poria cocos)
Jiang Huang (Curcuma longa)
Hou Pou (Magnolia officinalis)

Chen Pi (Citrus reticulata)
Zhi Ke (Citrus aurantium)
Chen Xiang (Aquilaria agallocha)
Mu Xiang (Saussurea lappa)
Chuan Lian Zi (Melia toosendan)
Dou Kou Ren (Amomum cardomomum)
Sha Ren (Amomum villosum)

Shu Gan
Yu Jin (Curcuma)
Chen Xiang (Aquilaria)
Yan Hu Suo (Corydalis)
Mu Xiang (Saussurea)
Rou Dou Kou (Nutmeg)
Bai Shao (White Peony)
Zhi Ke (Citrus Fruit)
Chen Pi (Citrus Peel)
Sha Ren (Cardamom)
Hou Po (Magnolia)
Xiang Fu (Cyperi)
Gan Cao (Licorice)
Dan Pi (Moutan)
Qing Pi (Immature Citrus Peel)
Tan Xiang (Sandalwood)

Xiao Chai Hu Tang (Minor Bupleurum Combination)
Bupleurum (Chai Hu)
Scutelleria (Huang Qin)
Pinellia Tuber (Ban Xia)
Fresh Ginger (Sheng Jiang)
Panax Ginseng (Ren Shen)
Licorice (Gan Cao)
Jujube (Da Zao)

Xiao Yao San
Chai Hu (Bupleurum chinense)
Dang Gui (Angelica sinensis)
Bai Shao Yao (Paeonia lactiflora)
Bai Zhu (Atractylodes macrocephala)
Fu Ling (Poria cocos)

Bo He (Mentha)
Sheng Jiang (Zingiberis officinale)
Gan Cao (Glycyrrhiza uralensis)

FOR CHRONIC HEPATITIS ADD:
Qian Cao Gen (Rubia cordifola)
Hai Piao Xiao (Sepiella maindroni)
Dang Shen (Codonopsis pilosula)

Woman's Balance (Health Concerns)
Chai Hu (Bupleurum chinense)
Dang Gui (Angelica sinensis)
Bai Shao (Paeonia lactiflora)
Dan Shen (Salvia miltorrhiza)
Fu Ling (Poria cocos)
Bai Zhu (Atractylodes)
Xiang Fu (Cyperus rotunda)
Chen Pi (Citrus reticulata)
Mu Dan Pi (Moutan radicis)
Zhi Zi (Gardenia jasminoides)
Gan Jiang (Zingiberis officinale, cooked)
Gan Cao (Glycyrrhiza)

Wei Ling Tang
Ze Xie (Alismatis plantago)
Fu Ling (Poria cocos)
Zhu Ling (Polyporus unbellatus)
Gui Zhi (Cinnamomum cassia)
Bai Zhu (Atractylodes macrocephala)
Cang Zhu (Atractylodes lancea)
Hou Po (Magnolia officinalis)
Chen Pi (Citrus reticulata)
Gan Cao (Glycyrrhiza)
Sheng Jiang (Zingiberis officinale)
Da Zao (Zizyphus jujube)

Channel Flow (Health Concerns)
Yan Hu Suo (Corydalis)
Bai Zhi (Angelica duhuo)
Bai Shao (White Peony)
Gui Zhi (Cinnamon Twig)

Dang Gui (Angelica sinensis)
Dan Shen (Salvia)
Mo Yao (Myrrh)
Ru Xiang (Frankincense)
Gan Cao (Licorice)

Li Gan Pian (Zhengjiang Chinese Medicine Works)
Jin Qian Cao (Lysimachia christinae)
Dan Zhi (Selenarctos thibetanus)

HERBAL FORMULAS FOR DAMP COLD

Wei Ling Tang (see page 278)

Shen Ling (Health Concerns)
Codonopsis (Dang Shen)
Atractylodes (Bai Zhu)
Poria (Fu Ling)
Baked Licorice (Zhi Gan Cao)
Dioscorea (Shan Yao)
Dolichosis (Bai Bian Dou)
Lotus Seed (Lian Zi)
Semen Coix (Yi Yi Ren)
Cardamom (Sha Ren)
Platycodon (Jie Geng)
Citrus Peel (Chen Pi)

Shen Ling (Shen Ling Bai Zhu San)
Ren Shen (Panax ginseng)
Bai Zhu (Rhizoma atractylodis macrophalae)
Shi Gan Cao (honey-fried radix glycyrrhizae uralensis)

Shan Yao (Radix dioscorea)
Bai Bian Dou (Semen dolichoris lablab)
Lian Zi (Semen nelumbinis nucifarae)
Sha Ren (Fructus amomi)
Jie Geng (Radix platycodi)
Fu Ling (Sclerotium poriae cocos)

Wu Ling San
Ze Xie (Alismatis)
Fu Ling (Poria)
Zhu Ling (Polyporus)
Gui Zhi (Cinnamon Twig)
Bai Zhu (White Atractylodes)

WHEN THERE IS ALSO JAUNDICE, WE ADD:
Yin Chen Hao (Artemesia capillaris), and then the formula is called *Yin Chen Wu Ling San.*

HERBAL FORMULAS FOR QI AND XUE DEFICIENCY

Ba Zhen Tang
Ren Shen (Panax Ginseng)
Shu Di Huang (Prepared Rehmannia)
Bai Zhu (White Atractylodes)
Dang Gui (Angelica sinensis)

Bai Shao (White Peony)
Chuan Xiong (Ligusticum)
Fu Ling (Poria)
Gan Cao (Licorice)
Sheng Jiang (Fresh Ginger)
Da Zao (Jujube Dates)

Eight Treasures (Health Concerns)
Codonopsis (Dang Shen)
Bai Zhu (Atractylodes)
Fu Ling (Poria)
Shu Di Huang (Rehmannia)
Bai Shao (Peony)
Dang Gui (Angelica sinensis)
Chuan Xiong (Ligusticum)
Ji Xue Teng (Spantholobus)
Zhi Gan Cao (Baked Licorice)
Gan Jiang (Ginger)
Da Zao (Red Dates)

Wu Ji Bai Feng Wan/Black Chicken White Phoenix Pills (Tientsin Drug Manufactory)
Wu Ji (Black Chicken)
Ren Shen (Panax Ginseng)
Huang Qi (Astragalus)
Dang Gui (Angelica sinensis)
Bai Shao (White Peony)
Sheng Di Huang (Raw Rehmannia)
Shu Di Huang (Prepared Rehmannia)
Xiang Fu (Cyperi)
Shan Yao (Dioscorea)
Lu Jiao Jiao (Deer Antler Glue)

Si Jun Zi Tang
Ren Shen (Panax Ginseng)
Bai Zhu (Atractylodes macrocephala)

Fu Ling (Poria cocos)
Gan Cao (Glycyrrhiza)

WITH QI STAGNATION ADD:
Chen Pi (Citrus reticulata)

WITH BLOOD DEFICIENCY ADD:
Si Wu Tang to make the formula *Ba Zhen Tang*

Si Wu Tang
Shu Di Huang (Rehmannia glutinosa, prepared)
Dang Gui (Angelica sinensis)
Chuan Xiong (Ligusticum wallichi)
Bai Shao (Paeonia lactiflora)

WITH QI DEFICIENCY ADD:
Si Jun Zi Tang to make the formula *Ba Zhen Tang*

WITH BLOOD (XUE) STAGNATION ADD:
Tao Ren (Semen persica)
Hong Hua (Carthamus tinctorius)

Xiao Yao San (see page 278)

Dan Zhi Xiao Yao San (see page 277)

Woman's Balance (see page 278)

HERBAL FORMULAS
FOR YIN DEFICIENCY

Yi Guan Jian
Shu Di Huang (Rehmannia glutinosa, raw)
Bai Sha Shen (Glehnia littoralis)
Mai Men Dong (Ophiopogon japonicus)

Dang Gui (Angelica sinensis)
Gou Qi Zi (Lycium chinense)
Chuan Lian Zi (Melia toosendan)

ADD FOR BITTER AND DRY MOUTH:
Huang Lian (Coptis chinensis)

ADD FOR CONSTIPATION:

Gua Luo Ren (Trichosanthes kirilowii fruit)

ADD FOR HYPOCHONDRIAC PAIN AND
HARD LUMPS:

Bei Jia (Amida sinensis/Tortoise shell)

ADD FOR SEVERE ABDOMINAL PAIN:

Bai Shao (Paeonia lactiflora)
Gan Cao (Glycyrrhiza)

HERBAL FORMULAS
FOR HEAT

Coptis Purge Fire (see page 277)   *Shen Ling Bai Zhu San (see page 279)*

APPENDIX III:
Liver-Toxic Medications and Herbs

There is a great deal of research still to be done to identify those prescription medications, over-the-counter drugs, herbs, and chemicals that are liver toxic. Some substances affect everyone negatively; some are dangerous for people who have liver disease. Others are hazardous when taken in too large a quantity, in combination with other substances, or by people who have unusual immune responses.

The following list of suspected or confirmed liver-toxic medications and herbs should help guide anyone with hepatitis. It is not comprehensive, however, and any time a person with liver disease contemplates taking a drug or herb, even when prescribed by a health-care practitioner, he or she should be on the lookout for negative reactions. Combining herbs with interferon and/or ribavirin demands particular care. Anyone with HCV should discuss potential reactions and drug interactions with both Western and Chinese medicine practitioners before taking any medication or herbal remedy. Although liver-toxic substances are identifiable in the laboratory, liver hypersensitivity problems are not predictable. In some cases, hypersensitivity may result in organ failure. Although hypersensitivity is hard to anticipate, there are some indicators that offer clues as to who may be vulnerable. Indicators of possible negative reactions to medical substances include:

- having multiple allergies and having had previous adverse reactions to drugs or herbs
- a history of chronic skin rashes
- current liver disease

Important: You should discontinue taking any drug or herb if you experience a skin rash, substantial nausea, bloating, fatigue and/or aching in the area of the liver, yellowing of the skin, or pale feces.

Dr. Gish has contributed information on liver-toxic drugs.

David L. Diehl, M.D., F.A.C.P., an associate clinical professor of medicine at UCLA School of Medicine, focuses on herbal toxicity. He, Ken Flora of the University of Oregon Health Sciences Center, and Misha Cohen are currently undertaking an extensive survey of the literature concerning the liver toxicity of herbal medicines.

PRESCRIPTION AND OVER-THE-COUNTER DRUGS

Patients who take the following medications regularly should undergo monthly laboratory testing for the first three months and then every three to six months to check on changes in liver function. Sample brand names are listed after the pharmaceutical name. Other products in addition to those mentioned may contain these drugs. Talk with your doctor and read all package inserts carefully.

acetaminophen (Tylenol), particularly hazardous when taken with alcohol or anti-seizure medications

alpha-methyldopa (Aldomet)

amiodarone (Cordarone)

carbamazapine (Atretol, Carbatrol)

chlorzoxazone (Parfon Forte DSC, Paraflex, Chlorzone Forte, Algisin)

dantrolene (Dantrium)

diclofenac (Voltaren, Cataflam)

fluconazole or ketoconazole (Diflucan, Nizoral)

flutamide (Drogenil)

hydralazine (Apresoline, Novo-Hylazin)

ibuprofen (Motrin)

azathioprine (Imuran, 6 mercaptopurine 6-MP)

isoniazid (INH) (Laniazid, Nydrazid)

long-acting nicotinic acid

luekotriene synthase inhibitors (Zafirlukast, Accolate and Zileuton, Zyflo) asthma medications

methotrexate (Maxtrex)

nitrofurantoin (Macrodantin)

PEXSIG (perhexiline maleate)

phenylbutazone (Mapap, Marnal, Lanatuss)

phenytoin (Ethotoin, Mephenytoin, Phenytoin)

pravastatin, fluvastatin, simavastatin, lovastatin

quinidine (Cardoquin, Cin-Quin, Duraquin)

rifampin (for TB)

sulfa medications (especially Septra or Bactrim)

tacrine (Cognex)

Tasmar (Tolcapone) for Parkinson's disease

ticlid (Ticlopidine)

troglitzone (Rezulin)

vitamin A (in doses greater than 5,000 units a day. Beta-carotene is safe at all doses)

According to an article published in the April 1996 *New England Journal of Medicine,* the most common cause of acute liver failure in the United States is the negative interaction between acetaminophen (Tylenol) and alcohol. Acetaminophen is one of the most commonly used over-the-counter drugs, either by itself, or used in combination with other drugs. It is used for pain, inflammation, and fever. Medical practitioners recommend it based largely on its great safety profile. The threshold of acetaminophen toxicity is lowered in people who drink alcohol moderately every day. If the liver is metabolizing alcohol and acetaminophen at the same time, the alcohol preoccupies the liver's detoxifying functions, making lower-than-usual intakes of acetaminophen toxic. This is called alcohol-acetaminophen syndrome. Liver toxicity can be seen with as little as 4 grams (eight 500 mg).

A 2006 study published in the *Journal of the American Medical Association* reported that healthy adults who took the maximum recommended dose of acetaminophen for two weeks had drastically increased liver enzyme levels that could lead to liver damage. Based on this research, the American Liver Foundation recommends "that people not exceed three grams of acetaminophen a day for any prolonged period of time. . . . This is the equivalent of six 'extra-strength' tablets a day for several weeks. Regular, short-term use of the product is not an issue. Anyone currently suffering from liver disease should check with their physician or hepatologist before taking acetaminophen."

In addition, there are interactions that are less common but equally as serious. Research suggests individual genetic variations in liver enzymes may be the cause.

CHINESE HERBAL PREPARATIONS

Herbal patent medicines, tonics, elixirs, and prepackaged solutions are particularly risky for anyone, whether or not they have liver disease. Ingredient labels may be incomplete or mistranslated. Herbs may be mistakenly used in the concoctions that are dangerous or inappropriate in combination with other herbs. Toxic herbs may be substituted for beneficial ones. The best bet is to avoid self-prescribed premixed preparations. Rely on the best-trained and most experienced herbalist available to individualize your herbal therapy and to monitor your reactions.

Some reportedly hazardous herbs and herb formulas:

Shosaikoto—a Japanese preparation used for improving hepatic dysfunction in chronic hepatitis. Its Chinese name is Xiao Chai Hu Tang. It may trigger interstitial pneumonia in people with chronic HCV who also are taking interferon, according to *Precautions* from the Pharmaceutical Affairs Bureau.

Jin Bu Huan—for insomnia and pain. This formula caused some liver problems but the exact trigger was never identified.

Aristolochia—used to treat fluid retention and rheumatic symptoms; has been banned in England after it was confused with an herb from the clematis plant that has the same name in Chinese as aristolochia: Mu Tong. The Mu Tong used was in fact the toxic species aristolochia, rather than the other, harmless herb. Aristolochia was part of a formula implicated in seventy cases of kidney failure in Belgium in 1993.

In addition, some Chinese patent medicines may contain heavy metals, poisons, and other potentially liver-toxic substances. In other cases, patent medicines contain Western pharmaceutical agents that are not listed on the label.

COMMON TOXIC INGREDIENTS FOUND IN ASIAN PATENT MEDICINES:

Be on guard for these ingredients:

aconite or aconitum: causes paralysis and death if not highly processed before use
acorus: causes convulsions and death
borax: triggers severe kidney damage
borneol: triggers internal bleeding and death
cinnabar or calomel: a mercury compound
litharge and minium: contain lead oxide
myiabris: can trigger convulsions, vomiting and death
orpiment or realgar: contains arsenic
scorpion or buthus: causes paralysis of the heart and death
strychnos nux vomica or semen strychni: strychnine-containing seeds cause respiratory failure and death
toad secretion or bufonis: can paralyze heart muscle and lungs

TOXIC INDIVIDUAL HERBS

Dr. Diehl writes: "Herbal medicine is generally safe—safer than Western pharmaceuticals. There are certain plants that are highly toxic. The most common examples are those that contain pyrolizidine alkaloids." Those that contain alkaloids or that reportedly have triggered toxic reactions include the following:

Chaparral (creosote bush, greasewood)
Comfrey (if taken internally)
Crotalaria (Ye Bai He)
Eupatorium
Germander (This toxic herb is often substituted for skullcap, and skullcap is not toxic in well-formulated herbal remedies. However, always insist that any ingredient identified as skullcap be the genuine article and not germander.)
Groundsel (senecio longilobus)
Heliotropium
Mentha pulegium
Mistletoe
Pennyroyal (squawmint) oil or Hedeoma pulegoides

Sassafras
Senicio species

SPECIAL CASES

Licorice: A mainstay of Chinese formulas, licorice is used in very small quantities to balance herbal action and often appears as glycyrrhizin (licorice root). However, licorice produces well-documented side effects such as hyperaldosteronism (an increase in levels of the adrenal hormone aldosterone, triggering imbalance of electrolytes) when taken in doses of more than 50 grams a day or for six weeks or longer. However, no side effects have been seen in smaller doses over thirty days or in higher doses for a very short period of time.

Skullcap: also called scutellaria or scute, this herb is used in many formulas to good effect. However, it appears that the toxic substance germander often is substituted for skullcap in formulas without being properly identified. As a result, skullcap looks like the offending substance. Dr. Diehl found several mentions of skullcap toxicity in the literature, but those mentions may in fact refer to unidentified substitutions of germander. Further research is needed to clarify this. Until then, whenever skullcap appears in a formula, make sure that it, not germander, is in fact being used. If you cannot be sure, do not take the formula or herb.

Dr. Diehl has found one mention of toxicity in the literature for the following herbs. Further documentation of toxicity is needed.

Calliepsis laureola
Atractylis gunnifera
margosa oil
valerian (Valerian officinalis)

Glossary of Terms and Abbreviations

Acupuncture: the art and science of manipulating the flow of Qi and Xue through the body's channels, the invisible aqueduct system that transports the Essential Substances to the Organ Systems, tissues, and bones. Manipulation of the Qi and Xue is accomplished by the stimulation of specific acupuncture points along the channels where these Essential Substances flow close to the skin's surface.

Acute Hepatitis: hepatitis that lasts less than six months.

Alanine Aminotransferase (ALT) and **Aspartate Aminotransferase (AST):** liver enzymes used for amino acid metabolism; elevated levels in the blood system may indicate liver injury and HCV.

Albumin: a blood protein manufactured by the liver. It is an indicator of the liver's ability to produce proteins in general and is essential in maintaining healthy circulation. Albumin acts like a sponge to hold fluid, salt, and water within the blood vessels and may actually help maintain the structural integrity of the vessels themselves. If there is not sufficient albumin—as happens when the liver develops cirrhosis—fluid leaks out of the vessels, causing swelling in the ankles and feet.

Alkaline Phosphatase: a liver enzyme that is responsible for phosphorus metabolism and for delivering energy to the body's cells.

Alphafetoprotein (AFP): a blood test for cancer in cirrhosis patients.

Amino Acids: the building blocks of proteins.

Ammonia: a blood toxin. High blood levels indicate the liver is unable to clean dangerous toxins from the body.

Anemia: a condition caused by chronic low red blood cell levels, indicated by pallor and weakness.

Antisense Oligonucleotides: a form of antiviral that prevents amino acids from being assembled into viral proteins, thereby blocking viral replication and mutation.

Arthralgias: the aches and pains associated with inflammation in the joints, possibly caused by immune complex molecules.

Ascites: the accumulation of excess fluid that causes swelling in the abdominal cavity.

Aspartate Aminotransferase (AST): see **Alanine Aminotransferase.**

Bacterial Peritonitis: a potential complication of HCV; it occurs when fluids become infected, causing abdominal pain and discomfort.

B-cell Non-Hodgkin's Lymphoma: a type of lymph node tumor or a cancer of the lymphatic system that is not Hodgkin's.

Bilirubin: a waste product that comes from a breakdown of heme, the central oxygen-carrying molecule in red blood cells. If not converted into a water-soluble substance by the liver, this yellowish liquid can act as a toxin, producing jaundice—the most vivid symptom of hepatitis.

Cerebral Vasculitis: inflammation of blood vessels in the brain.

Channels (also called **vessels** and **meridians**): the conduits that transport the Essential Substances to the Organ Systems. They contain the acupoints that are stimulated through acupuncture and acupressure.

Chronic Hepatitis: hepatitis that lasts more than six months.

Cirrhosis: severe liver disease characterized by extensive liver cell death and fibrosis.

Combination Therapy: treatment for hepatitis that includes the combination of interferon and ribavirin.

Corticosteroid: a hormone released into the blood system by the adrenal glands in response to perceived stress.

Cryoglobulinemia: inflammation caused by antibody-type proteins in the blood (serum) directed against HCV. They can gel or clump at low temperatures and cause a number of harmful side effects to the skin, kidney, eye, brain, and heart. A purplish or blue indicator on the skin where bleeding (ruptured blood vessels) has occurred is called purpura. Damage to the extremities—nose, ears, hands, and feet—from poor blood flow causes red feet and "red hands," or Raynaud's disease. A clustering or blocking of blood vessels in the kidneys causes glomerulonephritis. This can lead to kidney failure, dialysis, and transplantation.

Cytokines: immune system T cells produced by the thymus gland that battle viral infections.

Cytomegalovirus: a herpes virus that is an opportunistic infection associated with HIV/AIDS. It can lead to retinitis, blindness, colitis, pneumonia, and esophagitis.

Disharmony: an imbalance and improper functioning of the Essential Substances, Organ Systems, and/or channels. It can be created by the six Pernicious Influences or the seven Emotions.

Eight Fundamental Patterns of Disharmony: the ways in which the Pernicious Influences and seven Emotions create an imbalance in the mind/body/spirit. They are Interior, Exterior, Heat, Cold, Excess, Deficiency, Yin, and Yang.

ELISA II: a blood test that looks for the presence of antibodies to HCV.

Encephalopathy: a state of mental confusion or drowsiness caused by toxic elements in the blood (sometimes ammonia) that the HCV-infected liver is unable to clean.

Enzyme Immunoassay Tests (EIAs): methods of detecting antibodies against the virus containing HCV antigens.

Essential Substances: fluids, essences, and energies that nurture the Organ Systems and keep the mind/body/spirit in balance. They are identified as Qi, the life force; Shen, the mind-spirit; Jing, the essence that nurtures growth and development; Xue, which is often translated as blood but contains more qualities than blood, and transports Shen; and Jin-Ye, which is all the fluids not included in Xue.

Fetor Hepatiticus: having the smell of hepatitis, possibly detectable on the breath.

Fibrinogen: a protein used to control blood clotting.

Fibrosis: scar tissue in the liver that may be caused by chronic hepatitis.

Fibromyalgia (fibrositis): aches, pains, and stiffness between joints (bones) and the fibrous connective tissues (ligaments) of muscles. It may be an early warning sign of hepatitis.

Fulminant Hepatitis: acute hepatitis with liver failure.

Gamma-Glutamyltranspeptidase, or **GGT:** an enzyme used to metabolize the amino acid glutamate, which affects tissue oxidation.

Gastric Esophageal Variceal Bleeding: a life-threatening condition sometimes brought on by portal hypertension (restricted blood flow through the liver) where blood vessels in the esophagus or stomach rupture. The bleeding is difficult to stop, and surgery to repair the rupture is also life-threatening.

Glomerulonephritis: a condition associated with immune complexes—large, clumped-together molecules. They block vessels in the kidney, cause inflammation, and may lead to kidney failure.

HCV RNA: Hepatitis C virus ribonucleic acid.

Heme: the central oxygen-carrying molecule in red blood cells.

Hepatic Artery: an extension of the aorta that supplies the liver with oxygenated blood.

Hepatic Vein: a vessel that transports deoxygenated blood from the liver back to the heart.

Hepatitis: inflammation of the liver.

Hepatocellular Carcinoma: also called HCC, it is the medical terminology for liver cancer.

Hepatocytes: liver cells.

Hyperthyroidism: the elevated production of thyroid hormones.

Hypothyroidism: the lowered production of thyroid hormones.

INR Test: a composite method of evaluating the overall clotting function of at least five clotting factors.

Interferon: an antiviral protein that is a naturally occurring immune system response; it "interferes" with the viral replication of infected cells, hence, its name.

Jaundice: the yellowish pallor of the skin that results from the liver's inability to process bilirubin.

Jing: the fluid that nurtures growth and development; it is often translated as essence. We are born with Prenatal or Congenital Jing, inherited from our parents, and along with Original Qi, it defines our basic constitution.

Jin-Ye: all fluids other than Xue, including sweat, urine, mucus, saliva, bile, and gastric acid. It is produced by the digestion of food. Organ Qi regulates it. Certain forms of what is called "refined" Jin-ye help produce Xue.

Leukocytoclastic Vasculitis: tissue damage—a raised red and purple rash—due to ruptured blood vessels caused by cryoglobulinemia.

Lichen Planus: a dermatological disorder generally attributed to liver dysfunction. It is characterized by groups of small and irregular bumps with flat-topped surfaces that usually appear on the wrists, shins, lower back, and genital areas.

Liver Biopsy: the process whereby a small piece of the liver is surgically removed for clinical study. It is considered the gold standard in diagnosing hepatitis C, and does not affect liver function.

Monotherapy: drug treatment for hepatitis using only interferon.

Moxibustion: the use of burning herbs, placed on or near the body, to stimulate specific acupuncture points and warm the channels. It is used to stimulate a smooth flow of Qi and Xue.

Neuropathy: a nerve disease that triggers pain or numbness, usually in the feet or hands.

Nucleoside analogue: a type of antiviral medication that blocks the virus's ability to replicate and may alter the immune system cells that fight viruses, making them more effective. Ribavirin is a nucleoside analogue.

Organ System: the Chinese medicine concept in which an organ also includes its interaction with the Essential Substances and channels. For example, the Heart Organ System is responsible not only for what Western medicine calls the circulation of blood but also for the ruling of Xue and the storing of Shen.

Pegylated Interferon: a synthetic form of interferon in which polyethylene glycol molecules have been bound to the interferon molecule; pegylated interferon has a slower rate of breakdown and clearance from the body than standard interferon.

Pernicious Influences: Heat, Cold, Wind, Dampness, Dryness, and Summer Heat are associated with the development of disharmony and disease in the mind/body/spirit.

Polymerase Chain Reaction Assay Test (PCR): a method used to detect the RNA virus directly. The test measures viral load, that is, how many viruses exist in 1 milliliter of blood.

Porphyria Cutanea Tarda (PCT): a dermatological disorder generally attributed to "iron overload" found in several forms of chronic liver disease, including HCV.

Portal Hypertension: a condition that occurs in more than 65 percent of people with cirrhosis when pressure within the portal system increases to the point of causing inflammation. Collateral damage is most often found in the spleen, esophagus, and stomach.

Portal Vein: the major blood vessel responsible for two-thirds of the blood flow to the liver. This vein delivers both nutrients and toxins absorbed by the intestines to the liver for processing.

Protease Inhibitors: drugs that stop or inhibit protease enzymes from helping HIV to replicate.

Prothrombin: a protein used to control blood clotting.

Pruritis: itching of the skin that occurs when the liver cannot remove toxins from the blood and, consequently, the skin. Since antihistamines and lotions have no effect on pruritis caused by hepatitis, incapacitating pruritis can be reason enough for a liver transplant.

Purpura: a disease caused by blood leaking from blood vessels. It is characterized by purple or reddish brown spots on the skin and mucous membranes.

Qi: the basic life force that pulses through everything—living and inanimate. Qi warms the body, retains the body's fluids and organs, fuels the transformation of food into other substances such as Xue, protects the body from disease, and empowers movement—including physical movement, the movement of the circulatory system, thinking, and growth.

Qi Gong: the ancient Chinese art of exercise and meditation that stimulates and balances the mind/body/spirit.

Qi Gong Massage: an extension of Qi Gong exercise and meditation that also helps balance Qi and harmonize the mind/body/spirit.

Raynaud's Syndrome: a painful condition that can turn the nose, ears, hands, and feet a cold blue and sometimes white. It may result in severe skin damage.

Rebetron: the brand name of a combination of ribavirin and alpha interferon that is available from Schering-Plough.

Recombinant Immunoblot Assay Test (RIBA): a method of detecting antibodies against HCV antigens using an immunoblot format. It is less likely to give a false positive than ELISA.

Red Cell Hemolysis: a disease that breaks down red blood cells.

Reverse Transcription PCR (RT-PCR): generally accepted as the most sensitive test for detecting HCV.

Ribavirin: a nucleoside analogue used in combination therapy with interferon in the treatment of HCV.

Scleral Icterus: yellow eyes, indicating a buildup of bilirubin.

Seven Emotions: joy, anger, fear, fright, sadness, grief, and meditation, which are internal triggers of disharmony in mind/body/spirit.

Shen, or spirit: includes consciousness, thoughts, emotions, and senses that make us uniquely human. It is transmitted to the fetus from both parents and must be continuously nourished after birth.

Sinusoids: a system of small blood conduits that feed the hepatic artery and the portal vein.

Sodium Benzoate: a granular salt that absorbs ammonia in the intestines and carries it out of the body in the stools. It is sometimes used to treat encephalopathy.

Superinfection: the contraction of the hepatitis D virus by a person who already has the hepatitis B virus.

Tao: a philosophical concept and orientation (the word is sometimes translated as "the infinite origin" or the "Unnameable"), which underlies Chinese medicine's approach to healing, harmony, and wholeness. In the Tao there is no beginning and no end, yet whatever has a beginning has an end. Yin and Yang are the parts and the whole that epitomize the Tao of being.

Thyroiditis: inflammation of the thyroid that can result in hyper or hypothyroidism.

Vasculitis: a condition caused by inflammation of blood vessels.

Xue: an entity commonly translated as blood, but it is neither confined to the blood vessels, nor does it contain only plasma, red blood cells, and white blood cells. The Shen, or spirit, which courses through the blood vessels, is carried by Xue. Xue also moves along the channels in the body where Qi flows.

Yin and Yang: the dynamic balance between opposing forces, the ongoing process of creation and destruction, and the natural order of the universe and of each person's inner being.

Zinc Deficiency: a lack of the mineral zinc sometimes caused by liver disease; it can increase the amount of ammonia in the bloodstream.

Notes

CHAPTER 2: THE ABCs (AND BEYOND) OF HEPATITIS

1. P. B. Watkins; N. Kaplowitz; J. T. Slattery; C. R. Colonese; S. V. Colucci; P. W. Stewart; S. C. Harris; "Aminotransferase Elevations in Healthy Adults Receiving 4 Grams of Acetaminophen Daily: A Randomized Controlled Trial," *Journal of the American Medical Association* (2006) 296:87–93.
2. Centers for Disease Control and Prevention, www.cdc.gov
3. *MMWR*. Prevention of Hepatitis A Through Active or Passive Immunization: Recommendations of the Advisory Committee on Immunization Practices (ACIP); October 1, 1999 / 48(RR12);1–37
4. Ibid.
5. Ibid.
6. Ibid.
7. Australian Hepatitis Council, http://www.hepatitisaustralia.com/pages/About_the_Hepatitis_B_Virus.htm

CHAPTER 4: GETTING HIP TO HEPATITIS C

1. www.epidemic.org

CHAPTER 7: WESTERN DRUG THERAPY
FOR HEPATITIS C

1. *Archive of Virology* (1997) 142 (3): 535–44.
2. *Journal of Interferon Research* (1993) 13: 279–82.

CHAPTER 8: CHINESE HERBAL THERAPY FOR HEPATITIS C

1. G. Plomteaux, et al., "Hepatoprotector Action of Silymarin in Human Acute Viral Hepatitis," *IRCS Journal of Medical Science* (1979) 5:259.
2. *Chinese Medical Journal* (1981) 94 (1): 35–40; H. Yeung, *Handbook of Chinese Herbs and Formulas* (1985) 293.
3. *Chemical Abstract* 93:542y.

4. Ibid., 92: 51937t.

5. H. Kumanda, et al., "Study on Frequency of the eAg-eAb Seroconversion by Corticosteroid and Glycyrrhizin in eAg-Positive Chronic Hepatitis," *Nippon Shokakibyo Gakkai Zasshi* (Nov. 1981) 78 (11): 2195; H. Matsunami, et al., "Use of Glycyrrhizin for Recurrence of Hepatitis B After Liver Transplantation" (letter), *American Journal of Gastroenterology* (Jan. 1993) 88 (1): 152–53; W. Ohta, et al., "Treatment of Non-A, Non-B Hepatitis with Glycyrrhizin," Nippon Rinsho (Dec. 1988) 46(12): 2681–88; Z. H. Zhang et al., "Effect of Adenine-Arabinosine with Glycyrrhizin in Treating Chronic Active Hepatitis," *Chung Hsi I Chieh Ho Tsa Chih* (Mar. 1988) 8 (3):132–33, 150–51, 175.

6. Bensky and Gamble, *Chinese Herbal Medicine Materia Medica* (1933), Eastland Press (rev. ed.), 378.

7. Ibid.

8. H. Yeung (1985) 293.

9. Bensky and Gamble (1933) 269.

10. H. Yeung (1985) 125.

11. T. Ishizaki, et al., "Pneumanitis During Interferon and / or Herbal Drug Therapy in Patients with Chronic Active Hepatitis," *European Respiratory Journal* (Dec. 1991) 9 (12): 2691–6.

12. J. J. Carter, "Liver Protection and Repair: Synthesizing Herbal Science and Chinese Energetics," *Professional Health Concerns* 3 (1): 21–24.

13. Ibid.

CHAPTER 9. CHINESE NUTRITIONAL THERAPY

1. F. Corrao, P. A. Ferrari, and G. Galatola, "Exploring the Role of Diet in Modifying the Effect of Known Disease Determinants: Application to Risk Factors of Liver Cirrhosis," *American Journal of Epidemiology* (Dec. 1, 1995): 1136–46.

CHAPTER 10: RECIPES FOR A HEALTHY LIVER

1. www.soya.be/soy-thyroid.php

2. thyroid.about.com/gi/dynamic/offsite.htm?site=http//www.westonaprice.org/soy/darkside.html

CHAPTER 12. QI GONG: EXERCISE AND MEDITATION

1. "Stress and the Liver," *HCV Advocate* (April 2006) vol. 9 Alan Franciscus, pp44 source (source article: "Does Stress Exacerbate Liver Diseases?"; Y. Chida, N. Sudo, and C. Kubo. *Journal of Gastroenterology and Hepatology,* 20:202, 2006).

2. G. Abgrall-Barbry, and S. M. Consoli, "Psychological Approaches in Hypertension Management" (in French), *La Presse Medicale* (June 2006) 35 (6 pt. 2):1088–94.

3. W. E. Mehling, M. Acree, N. Byl, F. M. Hecht, "Randomized, Controlled Trial of Breath Therapy for Patients with Chronic Low-Back Pain," *Alternative Therapies in Health and Medicine* (July-Aug. 2005) 11 (4): 44–52.

4. H. Benson, H. P. Klemchuck, et al., "The Usefulness of the Relaxation Response in the Therapy of Headache," *Headache* (1974) 14 (1): 49–52.

5. J. A. Astin, S. L. Shapiro, D. M. Eisenberg, and K. L. Forys, "Mind-Body Medicine: State of the Science, Implications for Practice," *Journal of the American Board of Family Practice* (Mar.–Apr. 2003) 16 (2): 131–47.

6. H. Benson, F. H. Frankel, et al., "Treatment of Anxiety: A Comparison of the Usefulness of Self-Hypnosis and a Meditational Relaxation Technique. An Overview," *Psychotherapy and Psychosomatics* 30 (3–4): 229–42; J. K. Kempainen, L. S. Eller, E. Bunch, M. J. Hamilton, P. Dole, et al., "Strategies for Self-Management of HIV-Related Anxiety," *AIDS Care* (Aug. 2006) 18 (6): 597–607; T. Krisanaprakornkit, W. Krisanaprakornkit, N. Piyavhatkul, and M. Laopaiboon, "Meditation Therapy for Anxiety Disorders," *Cochrane Database of Systematic Reviews* (Jan. 25, 2006) (1): CD004998. Review.

7. S. M. Sagar, "Integrative Oncology in North America," *Journal of the Society for Integrative Oncology* (Wint. 2006) 4 (1): 27–39; M. J. Ott, R. L. Norris, and S. M. Bauer-Wu, "Mindfulness Meditation for Oncology Patients: A Discussion and Critical Review," *Integrative Cancer Therapies* (June 2006) 5 (2): 98–108.

8. V. B. Carson, "Prayer, Meditation, Exercise, and Special Diets: Behaviors of the Hardy Person with HIV/AIDS," *Journal of the Association of Nurses in AIDS Care* (July–Sept. 1993) 4 (3): 18–28; J. Barroso, "Self-Care Activities of Long-Term Survivors of Acquired Immunodeficiency Syndrome," *Holistic Nursing Practice* (Oct. 1995) 10 (1): 44–53; A. Mulkins, J. M. Morse, and A. Best, "Complementary Therapy Use in HIV/AIDS," *Canadian Journal of Public Health* (July–Aug. 2002) 93 (4): 308–12.

CHAPTER 16. IMMUNE-STRENGTHENING PROGRAM

1. Bandi, J. C., et al., "Effects of Propranolol on the Hepatic Hemodynamic Response to Physical Exercise in Patients with Cirrhosis," *Hepatology* (Sept. 1998) 28 (3): 677–82; Carl L. Berg and Fiona M. Graeme-Cook, "Exercise, Immunity, and Infection," *Journal of the American Osteopath Association* (Mar. 1996) 96 (3): 166–76.

CHAPTER 17. RELIEVING DEPRESSION AND FUZZY THINKING

1. "Double-Blind Placebo-Controlled Study of Gingko Biloba Extract in Elderly Outpatients with Mild to Moderate Memory Impairment," *Current Medical Research Opinion* (1991) 12: 350–55.

Background Sources

ABBREVIATIONS

Am J Epidemiol	American Journal of Epidemiology
Am J Gastroenterol	American Journal of Gastroenterology
Am J Med	American Journal of The Medical Sciences
Am J Pub Health	American Journal of Public Health
Ann Intern Med	Annals of Internal Medicine
Br J Ophthalmol	British Journal of Ophthalmology
Curr Med Res Opin	Current Medical Research and Opinion
Dig Dis Sci	Digestive Diseases and Sciences
Exerc Immunol Rev	Exercise Immunology Review
Gastroenterol Clin North Am	Gastroenterology Clinics of North America
J Clin Epidemiol	Journal of Clinical Epidemiology
J Clin Microbiol	Journal of Clinical Microbiology
J Gastroenterol Hepatol	Journal of Gastroenterology & Hepatology
J Hepatol	Journal of Hepatology
J Infect Dis	Journal of Infesctious Diseases
J Infect	Journal of Infection
J Med Virol	Journal of Medical Virology
J Natl Cancer Inst	Journal of the National Cancer Institute
J Am Osteopath Assoc	Journal of the American Osteopathic Association
J Rheumatol	Journal of Rheumatology
J Viral Hepat	Journal of Viral Hepatitis
J Virol	Journal of Virology
JAMA	Journal of the American Medical Association
Med Clin North Am	Medical Clinics of North America
Med Hypotheses	Medical Hypotheses
Med Sci Sports Exerc	Medicine and Science in Sports and Exercise
MMWR	Morbidity and Mortality Weekly Report
N Eng J Med	New England Journal of Medicine
Pediatr Infect Dis J	Pediatric Infectious Disease Journal
Proc Natl Acad Sci USA	Proceedings of the National Academy of Sciences of the United States of America
Prog Liver Dis	Progress in Liver Diseases
Scand J Gastroenterol	Scandinavian Journal of Gastroenterology

Sem Dialysis   *Seminars in Dialysis*
Semin Gastro Dis   *Seminars in Gastrointestinal Disease*
Semin Liver Dis   *Seminars in Liver Disease*
Semin Pediatr Inf Dis   *Seminars in Pediatric Infectious Diseases*

CHAPTER 2: THE ABCs (AND BEYOND) OF HEPATITIS

Advisory Committee on Immunization Practices (ACIP). Vaccines for Children
    Program: Resolution No. 10/97-1. Adopted October 23, 1997, Effective March 1,
    1998.
Centers for Disease Control and Prevention. Protection against viral hepatitis: Rec-
    ommendations of the Advisory Committee on Immunization Practices (ACIP).
    MMWR 1990;39:5–22.
Centers for Disease Control and Prevention. Hepatitis B virus: A comprehensive
    strategy for eliminating transmission in the United States through Universal Child-
    hood Vaccination. *MMWR* 1991;40 (RR-13):1–17.
Centers for Disease Control and Prevention. Immunization of adolescents: Recom-
    mendations of Advisory Committee on Immunization Practices, American Acad-
    emy of Pediatrics, American Family Physicians and American Medical Association.
    MMWR 1996; 45 (RR-13):1–14.
Centers for Disease Control and Prevention. Update on Adult Immunization: Rec-
    ommendations of the Immunization Practices Advisory Committee (ACIP).
    MMWR 1991;40 (RR-12);30–33.
Chen D. S. Control of hepatitis B in Asia: mass immunization program in Taiwan.
    In: Hollinger F.B., S. M. Lemon, H. S. Margolis, eds. Viral hepatitis and liver dis-
    ease. Baltimore: Williams and Wilkins, 1991:716–719.
Chen R. T., S. C. Rastogi, J. R. Mullen, S. Hayes, S. L. Cochi, J. A. Donlon, and
    S. G. Wassilak. The Vaccine Adverse Event Reporting System (VAERS). *Vaccine*
    1994;12:542–50.
Greenberg, D. P. "Pediatric Experience with Recombinant Hepatitis B Vaccines and
    Relevant Safety and Immunization Studies." *Pediatr Infect Dis J.* 1993;12:438–445.
Hadler, S. C., and H. S. Margolis. Hepatitis B Immunization: vaccine types, efficacy,
    and indications for immunization. In: Remington J. S., and M. N. Swartz, eds.
    "Current Clinical Topics in Infectious Diseases." Boston, Mass.: Blackwell Scien-
    tific Publications; 1992:282–308.
Kiely, J. National Center for Health Statistics, Presentation at the Vaccine Safety
    Forum October 26, 1998, Washington, D.C.
MMWR WEEKLY, Prevention of Hepatitis A Through Active or Passive Immu-
    nization: Recommendations of the Advisory Committee on Immunization Prac-
    tices (ACIP); October 01, 1999 / 48(RR12);1–37
Niu, M. T., D. M. Davis, S. Ellenberg. Recombinant hepatitis B vaccination of

neonates and infants: emerging safety data from the Vaccine Adverse Event Reporting System. *Pediatr Inf Dis J*, 1996;15:771–6.

Niu, M. T., P. Rhodes, M. Salive, T. Lively, et al. Comparative safety data of two recombinant hepatitis B vaccines in children: data from the Vaccine Adverse Event Reporting System (VAERS) and Vaccine Safety Datalink (VSD). *J Clin Epidemiol;* 1998;51:503–10.

Pope, J. E., S. Adams, W. Howson, et al. The development of rheumatoid arthritis after recombinant hepatitis b vaccination. *J Rheumatol;* 1998; 25: 1687–93.

Shaw F. E., D. J. Graham, H. A. Guess, et al. Postmarketing surveillance for neurologic adverse events reported after hepatitis B vaccination. *Am J Epidemiol* 1988; 127:337–352.

Sibley W. A., et al. Clinical viral infections and multiple sclerosis. *Lancet* 1985; 1:1313–1315.

Szmuness W., C. E. Stevens, E. J. Harley, et al. Hepatitis B vaccine: demonstration of efficacy in a controlled clinical trial in a high risk population in the United States. *N Engl J Med;* 1980; 303:833–841.

Watkins P. B., N. Kaplowitz, J. Slattery, et al. Aminotransferase Elevations in Healthy Adults Receiving 4 Grams of Acetaminophen Daily: A Randomized Controlled Trial; *JAMA,* 2006;296:87–93.

West D. J., and H. S. Margolis. Prevention of hepatitis B virus infection in the United States: a pediatric perspective. *Pediatr Infect Dis J*, 1992;11:866–874.

Zajac B. A., D. J. West, W. J. McAleer, and E. M. Scolnick. Overview of clinical studies with hepatitis B vaccine made by recombinant DNA. *J Infect* 1986; 13(Suppl A):39–45.

CHAPTER 4: GETTING HIP TO HEPATITIS C

Alter, H. J. 1990. The Hepatitis C Virus and Its Relationship to the Clinical Spectrum of NANB Hepatitis. *J Gastroenterol Hepatol* 5 (Suppl 1): 78–94.

Alter, M. J. 1991. Hepatitis C: A Sleeping Giant? *Am J Med;* 91:112S–15S.

Alter, M. J. 1993. Community-Acquired Viral Hepatitis B and C in the United States. *Gut;* 34 (Suppl 1):S17–19.

Alter, M. J. 1995. Epidemiology of Hepatitis C in the West. *Semin Liver Dis;* 15:5–14.

Alter, M. J., et al. 1990. Risk Factors for Acute Non-A, Non-B Hepatitis in the United States and Association with Hepatitis C Virus Infection. *JAMA* 264: 2231–35.

Alter, M. J., et al. 1992. The Natural History of Community-Acquired Hepatitis C in the United States. The Sentinel Counties Chronic Non-A, Non-B Hepatitis Study Team. *N Engl J Med* 327:1899–1905.

Bukh, J., R. H. Miller, and R. H. Purcell. 1995. Genetic Heterogeneity of Hepatitis C Virus: Quasispecies and Genotypes. *Semin Liver Dis* 15:41–46.

Castilla, A., et al. 1993. Lymphoblastoid Alpha-Interferon for Chronic Hepatitis C: A Randomized Controlled Study. *Am J Gastroenterol* 88:233–39.

Choo, Q. L., et al. 1989. Isolation of a CDNA Clone Derived from a Blood-Borne Non-A, Non-B Viral Hepatitis Genome. *Science* 244:359–62.

Craxi, A., et al. 1994. Third-Generation Hepatitis C Virus Tests in Asymptomatic Anti-HCV-Positive Blood Donors. *J Hepatol* 21:730–34.

Davis, G. L. Interferon Treatment of Chronic Hepatitis C. *Am J Med* 96:41S–46S.

De Medina, M., and E. R. Schiff. 1995. Hepatitis C: Diagnostic Assays. *Semin Liver Dis* 15:33–40.

Di Bisceglie, A. M., et al. 1991. Long-term Clinical and Histopathological Follow-up of Chronic Post-transfusion Hepatitis. *Hepatology* 14:969–74.

Esteban, J. I., J. Genesca, and H. J. Alter. 1992. Hepatitis C: Molecular Biology, Pathogenesis, Epidemiology, Clinical Features, and Prevention. *Prog Liver Dis* 10:253–82.

Farci, P., et al. 1992. Lack of Protective Immunity Against Reinfection with Hepatitis C Virus. *Science* 258:135–40.

Farci, P., et al. 1994. Prevention of Hepatitis C Virus Infection in Chimpanzees After Antibody-Mediated In-Vitro Neutralization. *Proc Natl Acad Sci USA* 91: 7792–96.

Fried, M. W., and J. H. Hoofnagle. 1995. Therapy of Hepatitis C. *Semin Liver Dis* 15:82–91.

Garcia-Samaniego, J., et al. 1994. Hepatitis B and C Virus Infections Among African Immigrants in Spain. *Am J Gastroenterol* 89:1918–19.

Han, J. H., et al. 1991. Characterization of the Terminal Regions of Hepatitis C Viral RNA: Identification of Conserved Sequences in the 5 Untranslated Region and Poly(A) Tails at the 3 End. *Proc Natl Acad Sci USA* 88:1711–15.

Hino, K., et al. 1994. Genotypes and Titers of Hepatitis C Virus for Predicting Response to Interferon-Alfa. *J Med Virol* 42: 299–305.

Kato, N., et al. 1990. Molecular Cloning of the Human Hepatitis C Virus Genome from Japanese Patients with Non-A, Non-B Hepatitis. *Proc Natl Acad Sci USA* 87:9524–28.

Kobayashi, Y., et al. 1993. Quantitation and Typing of Serum Hepatitis C Virus RNA in Patients with Chronic Hepatitis C Treated with Interferon-Beta. *Hepatology* 18:1319–25.

Konishi, M. 1994. Titration and Genotyping of Hepatitis C Virus RNA in Chronic Hepatitis C Patients Treated with Interferon. *Nippon Shokakibyo Gakkai Zasshi* 91:147–53.

Kuo, G., et al. 1989. An Assay for Circulating Antibodies to a Major Etiologic Virus of Human Non-A, Non-B Hepatitis. *Science* 244:362–64.

Mansell, C. J., and S. A. Locarnini. 1995. Epidemiology of Hepatitis C in the East. *Semin Liver Dis* 15:15–32.

Marcellin, P., et al. 1991. Second-Generation (RIBA) Test in Diagnosis of Chronic Hepatitis C. *Lancet* 337:551–52.

Matsumoto, A., et al. 1994. Vital and Host Factors That Contribute to Efficacy of Interferon-Alpha 2a Therapy in Patients with Chronic Hepatitis C. *Dig Dis Sci* 39:1273–80.

Mattsson, L., et al. 1991. Antibodies to Recombinant and Synthetic Peptides Derived from the Hepatitis C Virus Genome in Long-Term-Studied Patients with Post-transfusion Hepatitis C. *Scand J Gastroenterol* 26:1257–62.

Mattsson, L., O. Weiland, and H. Glaumann. 1988. Long-term Follow-up of Chronic Post-Transfusion Non-A, Non-B Hepatitis: Clinical and Histological Outcome. *Liver* 184–88.

Mita, E., et al. 1994. Predicting Interferon Therapy Efficacy from Hepatitis C Virus Genotype and RNA Titer. *Dig Dis Sci* 39:977–82.

Osmond, D. H., et al. 1993. Risk Factors for Hepatitis C Virus Seropositivity in Heterosexual Couples. *JAMA* 269:361–65.

Seeff, L. B., et al. 1992. Long-term Mortality After Transfusion-Associated Non-A, Non-B Hepatitis. The National Heart, Lung, and Blood Institution Study Group. *N Engl J Med* 327:1906–11.

Shimizu, Y. K., et al. 1994. Neutralizing Antibodies Against Hepatitis C Virus and the Emergence of Neutralization Escape Mutant Viruses. *J Virol* 68:1494–1500.

Takahashi, M., et al. 1993. Natural Course of Chronic Hepatitis C. *Am J Gastroenterol* 88:240–43.

Tremolada, F., et al. 1992. Long-term Follow-up of Non-A, Non-B (Type C) Post-Transfusion Hepatitis. *J Hepatol* 16:273–81.

Tsubota, A., et al. 1993. Factors Useful in Predicting the Response to Interferon Therapy in Chronic Hepatitis C. *J Gastroenterol Hepatol* 8:535–39.

Tsubota, A., et al. 1994. Factors Predictive of Response to Interferon-Alpha Therapy in Hepatitis C Virus Infection. *Hepatology* 19:1088–94.

Weiner, A. J., et al. 1991. Variable and Hypervariable Domains Are Found in the Regions of HCV Corresponding to the Flavivirus Envelope and NS1 Proteins and the Pestivirus Envelope Glycoproteins. *Virology* 180:842–48.

Widell, A., et al. 1991. Hepatitis C Virus RNA in Blood Donor Sera Detected by the Polymerase Chain Reaction: Comparison with Supplementary Hepatitis C Antibody Assays. *J Med Virol* 35:253–58.

Natural History

Alter, M. J., et al. 1992. "The Natural History of Community-Acquired Hepatitis C in the United States." *N Engl J Med* 327:1899–1905.

Bellentani, S., et al. 1994. Prevalence of Chronic Liver Disease in the General Population of Northern Italy: The Dionysos Study. *Hepatology* 20:1442–49.

DeBac, C., et al. 1994. Pathogenic Factors in Cirrhosis with and Without Hepatocellular Carcinoma: A Multicenter Italian Study. *Hepatology* 20:1225–30.

Di Bisceghe, A. M., et al. 1991. The Role of Chronic Viral Hepatitis in Hepatocellular Carcinoma and Alcoholic Liver Disease. *Hepatology* 12:70–74.

Koff, R. S., and J. L. Dienstag. 1995. Extrahepatic Manifestations of Hepatitis C and the Association with Alcoholic Liver Disease. *Semin Liver Dis* 15:101–9.

Poynard, T., P. Bedossa, and P. Opolon. 1997. Natural History of Liver Fibrosis Progression in Patients with Chronic Hepatitis C. *Lancet* 1997; 349:825–32.

Seeff, L. B. 1995. Natural History of Viral Hepatitis, Type C. *Semin Gastro Dis* 6:20–27.

Shakil, A. O., et al. 1995. Volunteer Blood Donors with Antibody to Hepatitis C Virus: Clinical, Biochemical Virologic, and Histologic Features. *Ann Intern Med* 123:330–37.

Stroffolini, T., et al. 1992. Hepatitis C Virus Infection, HBsAg Carrier State and Hepatocellular Carcinoma: Relative Risk and Population Attributable Risk from a Case-control Study in Italy. *J. Hepatol* 16:360–63.

Yu, M. C., et al. 1990. Prevalence of Hepatitis B and C Viral Markers in Black and White Patients with Hepatocellular Carcinoma in the United States. *J. Natl Cancer Inst* 82:1038–41.

Disease Burden and Epidemiology

Aach, R. D., et al. 1991. Hepatitis C Virus Infection in Post-transfusion Hepatitis: An Analysis with First-and Second-Generation Assays. *N Engl J Med* 325:1325–29.

Alter, H. J., et al. 1989. Detection of Antibody to Hepatitis C Virus in Prospectively Followed Transfusion Recipients with Acute and Chronic Non-A, Non-B Hepatitis. *N Engl J Med* 321:1494–1500.

Alter, M. J. 1995. Epidemiology of Hepatitis C in the West. *Semin Liver Dis* 15:5–13.

Alter, M. J. 1997. The Epidemiology of Acute and Chronic Hepatitis C. *Liver Clinics of North America*, in press.

Bresee, J. S., et al. 1996. Hepatitis C Virus Infection Associated with Administration of Intravenous Immune Globulin. *JAMA* 276:1563–67.

Centers for Disease Control. 1997. Transmission of Hepatitis C Virus Infection Associated with Home Infusion Therapy for Hemophilia. *MMWR* 46: 597–99.

Conry-Cantilena, C., et al. 1996. Routes of Infection, Viremia, and Liver Disease in Blood Donors Found to Have Hepatitis C Virus Infection. *N Engl J Med* 334:1691–96.

Esteban, J. I., et al. 1995. Transmission of Hepatitis C Virus by a Cardiac Surgeon. *N Engl J Med* 334: 555–60.

Garfein R. S., et al. 1996. Viral Infections in Short-term Injection Drug Users: The Prevalence of the Hepatitis C, Hepatitis B, Human Immunodeficiency, and Human T-Lymphotropic Viruses. *Am J Pub Health* 86:655–61.

Mast, E. E., and M. J. Alter. 1997. Hepatitis C. *Semin Pediatr Inf Dis* 8:17–22.

Moyer, L. A., and M. J. Alter. 1994. Hepatitis C Virus in the Hemodialysis Setting: A Review with Recommendations for Control. *Sem Dialsis* 7:124–27.

Ohto, H., et al. 1994. Transmission of Hepatitis C Virus from Mothers to Infants. *N Engl J Med* 3310:744–50.

Schreiber, G. B., et al. 1996. The Risk of Transfusion-Transmitted Viral Infections. *N Engl J Med* 334:1685–90.

Seeff, L. B., and H. J. Alter. 1994. Spousal Transmission of the Hepatitis C Virus. *Ann Intern Med* 20:807–9.

Thomas, D. L., et al. 1995. Sexual Transmission of Hepatitis C Virus Among Patients Attending Baltimore Sexually Transmitted Diseases Clinics—an Analysis of 309 Sex Partnerships. *J Infect Dis* 171: 768–75.

Screening and Diagnostic Tests

DeMedina, M., and E. R. Schiff. 1995. Hepatitis C: Diagnostic Assays. *Semin Liver Dis* 15:33–40.

National Institutes of Health. 1997. National Institutes of Health Consensus Development Conference Panel Statement: Management of Hepatitis C. *Hepatology* 26:2S–10S.

Prevention and Counseling

American Academy of Pediatrics. 1997. Hepatitis C. In: Peter G., ed., *1997 Red Book: Report of the Committee on Infectious Diseases, 24th ed.* Elk Grove Village, Ill.: American Academy of Pediatrics, pp.260–65.

Centers for Disease Control. 1991. Hepatitis B Virus: A Comprehensive Strategy for Eliminating Transmission in the United States Through Universal Childhood Vaccination: Recommendations of the Immunization Practices Advisory Committee (ACIP). *MMWR* 40 (RR-13): 1–25.

Centers for Disease Control. 1996. Prevention of Hepatitis A Through Active or Passive Immunization: Recommendations of the Advisory Committee on Immunization Practices (ACIP). *MMWR* 45 (RR-15):1–30.

Centers for Disease Control. 1991. Public Health Service Inter-Agency Guidelines for Screening Donors of Blood, Plasma, Organs, Tissues, and Semen for Evidence of Hepatitis B and Hepatitis C. *MMWR* 40 (RR-4):1–17.

Centers for Disease Control. 1997. Recommendations for Follow-up of Health-Care Workers After Occupational Exposure to Hepatitis C Virus. *MMWR* 46:603–6.

Centers for Disease Control. 1997. Transmission of Hepatitis C Virus Infection Associated with Home Infusion Therapy for Hemophilia. *MMWR* 46:597–99.

Centers for Disease Control. HRSA, NIDA, SAMHSA. May 1997. Medical Advice for Persons Who Inject Illicit Drugs. *HIV Prevention Bulletin.*

Dusheiko, G. M., et al. 1996. A Rational Approach to the Management of Hepatitis C Infection. *BMJ* 312:357–64.

Gostin, L. O., et al. 1997. Prevention of HIV/AIDS and Other Blood-Borne Diseases Among Injection Drug Users: A National Survey on the Regulation of Syringes and Needles. *JAMA* 277:53–62.

Hagan, H., et al. 1995. Reduced Risk of Hepatitis B and Hepatitis C Among Injecting Drug Users Participating in the Tacoma Syringe Exchange Program. *Am J Pub Health* 85:1531–37.

Koester, S. K., and L. Hoffer. 1994. "Indirect Sharing": Additional HIV Risks Associated with Drug Injection. *AIDS and Pub Policy J* 9:100–5.

Krawczynski, K., et al. 1996. Effect of Immune Globulin on the Prevention of Experimental Hepatitis C Virus Infection. *J Infect Dis* 173:822–28.

Mast, E. E., and M. J. Alter. 1997. Hepatitis C. *Semin Pediatr Inf Dis* 8:17–22.

Miller, R. 1995. Guidelines for Counseling Adolescents with Hemophilia and HIV Infection and Their Families. *Aids Care* 7:381–89.

National Institutes of Health. 1997. National Institutes of Health Consensus Development Conference Panel Statement: Management of Hepatitis C. *Hepatology* 26:2S–10S.

Management and Treatment

Di Besceghe, A. M., et al. 1995. Ribavirin as Therapy for Chronic Hepatitis C. *Ann Intern Med* 123:897–903.

Fried, M. W. 1996. Therapy of Chronic Viral Hepatitis. *Med Clin of North Am* 80:957–72.

Hoofnagle, J. H., and A. M. Di Bisceghe. 1997. The Treatment of Chronic Viral Hepatitis. *N Engl J Med* 5:347–56.

National Institutes of Health. 1997. National Institutes of Health Consensus Development Conference Panel Statement: Management of Hepatitis C. *Hepatology* 26:2S–10S.

Poynard, T., et al. 1995. A Comparison of Three Interferon Alfa-2b Regimens for the Long-term Treatment of Chronic Non-A, Non-B Hepatitis. *N Engl J Med* 332:1457–62.

Poynard, T., et al. 1996. Meta-analysis of Interferon Randomized Trials in the Treatment of Viral Hepatitis C: Effects of Dose and Duration. *Hepatology* 24:778–89.

Schvarcz, R., et al. 1995. Combined Treatment with Interferon Alpha-2b and Ribavirin for Chronic Hepatitis C in Patients with a Previous Non-Response or Non-Sustained Response to Interferon Alone. *J Med Virol* 46:43–47.

CHAPTER 7: WESTERN DRUG THERAPY FOR HEPATITIS C

Aiyama, T., et al. 1995. Serum HCV RNA Titer at the End of Interferon Therapy Predicts the Long-term Outcome of Treatment. *J Hepatol* 23:497–502.

Bennett, W. G., et al. 1997. Estimates of the Cost-Effectiveness of a Single Course of Interferon-Alpha 2b in Patients with Histologically Mild Chronic Hepatitis C. *Ann Intern Med* 127(10):855–65.

Bortolotti, F., et al. 1990. Long-term Outcome of Chronic Type B Hepatitis in Patients Who Acquire Hepatitis B Virus Infection in Childhood. *Gastroenterology* 99(3):805–10.

Bossy, J. 1990. Immune Systems, Defense Mechanisms and Acupuncture: Fundamental and Practical Aspects. *American Journal of Acupuncture* 18(3).

Hawkins, A., F. Davidson, and P. Simmonds. 1997. Comparison of Plasma Virus Loads Among Individuals Infected with Hepatitis C Virus (HCV) Genotypes 1, 2, and 3 by Quantiplex HCV RNA Assay Versions 1 and 2, Roche Monitor Assay, and an In-house Limiting Dilution Method. *J Clin Microbiol* 35: 187–92.

Hollingsworth, R. C., et al. 1996. Serum HCV RNA Levels Assessed by Quantitative NASBA: Stability of Viral Load over Time, and Lack of Correlation with Liver Disease. The Trent HCV Study Group. *J Hepatol* 25:301–6.

Kakumu, S., et al. 1997. Earlier Loss of Hepatitis C Virus RNA in Interferon Therapy Can Predict a Long-term Response in Chronic Hepatitis C see comments. *J Gastroenterol Hepatol* 12:468–72.

Romeo, R., et al. 1996. Lack of Association Between Type of Hepatitis C Virus, Serum Load and Severity of Liver Disease. *J Viral Hepat* 3:183–90.

Shiratori, Y., et al. 1997. Predictors of the Efficacy of Interferon Therapy in Chronic Hepatitis C Virus Infection. Tokyo-Chiba Hepatitis Research Group. *Gastroenterology* 113:558–66.

Stoll, Matthias, et al. July 1998. Response and Toxicity of Interferon (IFN) 2a Treatment in Chronic Hepatitis C (HCV) in HIV-Infected Patients, Poster 32116, 12th International AIDS Conference. Geneva, Switzerland.

Takase, S., et al. 1993. The Alcohol Altered Liver Membrane Antibody and Hepatitis C Virus Infection in the Progression of Alcoholic Liver Disease. *Hepatology* 17:9–13.

Thomas, D., et al. 1995. Correlates of Hepatitis C Infection in Injection Drug Users. *Medicine* 74(4): 212–20.

Trabaud, M. A., et al. 1997. Comparison of HCV RNA Assays for the Detection and Quantification of Hepatitis C Virus RNA Levels in Serum of Patients with Chronic Hepatitis C Treated with Interferon. *J Med Virol* 52:105–12.

Daily Interferon References

Bresters, D., et al. 1992. Disappearance of Hepatitis C Virus RNA in Plasma During Interferon Alpha-2B Treatment in Hemophilia Patients. *Scand J Gastroenterol* 27:166–68.

Carreno, V., et al. 1992. Treatment of Chronic Hepatitis C by Continuous Subcutaneous Infusion of Interferon-alpha. *J Med Virol* 37:215–19.

Chayama, K., et al. 1994. Antiviral Effect of Lymphoblastoid Interferon-alpha on Hepatitis C Virus in Patients with Chronic Hepatitis Type C. *J Gastroenterol Hepatol* 9:128–33.

Ferenci, P., et al. 1990. One-Year Treatment of Chronic Non-A, Non-B Hepatitis with Interferon Alfa J 2b. *J. Hepatol* 11 (Suppl 1): S50–S53.

Iino, S. 1993. High-dose Interferon Treatment in Chronic Hepatitis C. *Gut* 34: S114–18.

Iino, S., et al. 1993. Treatment of Chronic Hepatitis C with High-Dose Interferon Alpha-2b: A Multicenter Study. *Dig Dis Sci* 38:612–18.

Ohnishi, K., F. Nomura, and M. Nakano. 1991. Interferon Therapy for Acute Posttransfusion Non-A, Non-B Hepatitis: Response with Respect to Anti-hepatitis C Virus Antibody Status. *Am J Gastroenterol* 86:1041–49.

Saito, T., et al. 1994. A Randomized, Controlled Trial of Human Lymphoblastoid Interferon in Patients with Compensated Type C Cirrhosis. *Am J Gastroenterol* 89:681–86.

Shindo, M., A. M. Di Bisceghe, and J. H. Hoofnagle. 1992. Long-term Follow-up of Patients with Chronic Hepatitis C Treated with Interferon-Alfa. *Hepatology* 15:1013–16.

Shoji, S., et al. 1991. Clinical Study on Long-term Treatment of Chronic Hepatitis C with Interferon. *Nippon Shokakibyo Gakkai Zasshi* 88:706–13.

Tsubota, A., et al. 1993. Factors Useful in Predicting the Response to Interferon Therapy in Chronic Hepatitis C. *J Gastroenterol Hepatol* 8:535–39.

Yamada, G., et al. 1993. Quantitative Hepatitis C Virus RNA and Liver Histology in Chronic Hepatitis C Patients Treated with Interferon Alfa. *Gut* 34:S133–34.

CHAPTER 8: CHINESE HERBAL THERAPY FOR HEPATITIS C

Chen, N. L., F. Gu, and K. M. Jia. Mar. 1990. Chronic Active Hepatitis with Superinfection of Delta Virus and Hepatitis B Virus: Treatment with Traditional Chinese Medicine. *Chinese Journal of Internal Medicine* 29 (3):144–46, 189.

Chinese Medical Journal (1981) 94(1):35–40.

Cohen, M. 1990. Chinese Medicine in the Treatment of Chronic Immunodeficiency: Diagnosis and Treatment. *American Journal of Acupuncture* 18(2) 111–22.

Desheng, D. 1997. 30 Cases of Hepatitis C Treated with Song Zhi Mixture. *Hunan Journal of Traditional Chinese Medicine* 13(6):27–28.

Hougen, L., et al. 1994. Qingtui Fang Applied in Treating 128 Cases of Chronic Hepatitis C. *Chinese Journal of Integrated Traditional and Western Medicine for Liver Diseases* (5) 4(2):40.

Huiwen, H., et al. 1997. Analysis of Clinical and Therapeutic Specificity in Treating Chronic Hepatitis B and C. *Journal of Traditional Chinese Medicine* 38(12):732–34.

Ishizaki, T., et al. 1996. Pneumonitis During Interferon and/or Herbal Drug Therapy in patients with Chronic Active Hepatitis. *European Respiratory Journal* 9(12): 2691–6.

Jiawu, L. 1995. 32 Chronic Hepatitis C Patients Treated by Integrating Chinese Herbs and Interferon. *Chinese Journal of Integrated Traditional and Western Medicine* 15(6):371.

Lin, C. C., et al. 1990. The Pharmacological and Pathological Studies on Taiwan Folk Medicine (III): The Effects of Bupleurum Kaoi and Cultivated Bupleurum Falcatum var. Komarowi. *American Journal of Chinese Medicine* 18(3–4): 105–12.

Liu, K. June 10, 1990. Preliminary Report on Various Symptoms of Chronic Hepatitis Treated with Radix Astragali and Its Regulative Effect on Levels of Serum Hormone. *Chinese Journal of Modern Developments in Traditional Medicine* 10 (6):323, 330–33.

Magliulo, E., et al. 1973. "Studies on the Regenerative Capacity of the Liver in Rats Subjected to Partial Hepatectomy and Treated with Silymarin," *Arzneimittelforschung* 23:161–67.

Qingchi, L., et al. 1995. Clinical Study of Traditional Chinese Medicine and Western Medicine on Aplastic Anemia Complicated with Hepatitis C. *Chinese Journal of Traditional and Western Medicine* 15(4): 198–201.

Schopen, R., and O. Lang. 1971. "Therapy in H: Therapeutic Use of Silymarin," *Arzneimittelforschung* 21:1209–12.

Shi, J., and C. Quanliang. 1994. Clinical Manifestations of Hepatitis C and Hepatitis B: A Comparative Approach Utilizing TCM differential Diagnostics. *Journal of Traditional Chinese Medicine* (9).

Shi J., and W. Yue. 1998. Probing into the Relationship Between the TCM Differentiations of Chronic Hepatitis C and Clinical Determination Results. *Journal of Traditional Chinese Medicine* 39(4):233–35.

Velussi, M., et al. 1993. "Silymarin Reduces Hyperinsulinemia, Malodial-Dehyde Levels, and Daily Insulin Need in Cirrhotic Diabetes Patients," *Current Therapeutic Research* 53 (5):533–45.

Wang, C. B. Apr. 1992. Treatment of Severe Chronic Hepatitis B by Combination of Traditional Chinese Medicine and Western Medicine Therapy—with Analysis of 122 Cases. *Chung Kuo Chieh Ho Tsa Chin* (China) 12 (4):203–6, 195.

Wu, C., et al. 1994. 33 Patients with Hepatitis C Treated by TCM Syndrome Differentiation. *Chinese Journal of Integrated Traditional and Western Medicine for Liver Diseases* 4(1): 44–45.

Zhang, Y. Feb. 1990. Discussion on Some Aspects of Clinical Observation on Traditional Chinese Medicine Treatment of Viral Hepatitis. *Chinese Journal of Modern Developments in Traditional Medicine* 10 (2): 116–17.

Zhao, R., and H. Shen. 1991. Antifibrogenesis with Traditional Chinese Herbs. International Symposium on Viral Hepatitis and AIDS, Beijing, China. Sponsors: Beijing Association of Integration of Traditional and Western Medicine and China Medical Association. *Abstract,* p. 20.

Zhen, Y., L. Maocai, and W. Chaolian. 1995. A Preliminary Report on the Affect of 911 Granules on Chronic Viral Hepatitis of the B and C Types. *Journal of Integrated Traditional and Western Medicine* 3.

Zhou, I., et al. Jan. 1990. Short-term Curative Effects of Cultured Cordyceps Sinensis (Berk.) Secc. Mycelia in Chronic Hepatitis B. *China Journal of Chinese Materia Medica* 15 (1):53–55, 65.

CHAPTER 12: QI GONG: EXERCISE AND MEDITATION

Bandi, J. C., et al. Sept. 1998. Effects of Propranolol on the Hepatic Hemodynamic Response to Physical Exercise in Patients with Cirrhosis. *Hepatology* 28(3): 677–82.

Berg, Carl L., and Fiona M. Graeme-Cook. Mar. 1996. Exercise, Immunity, and Infection. *J Am Osteopath Assoc* 96(3):166–76.

Double-Blind Placebo-Controlled Study of Ginkgo Biloba Extract in Elderly Outpatients with Mild to Moderate Memory Impairment. 1991. *Curr Med Res Opin* 12:350–55.

Garcia-Pagan, J. C., et al. Nov. 1996. Physical Exercise Increases Portal Pressure in Patients with Cirrhosis and Portal Hypertension. *Gastroenterology* 111(5): 1300–6.

Glaser R., and J. K. Kiecolt-Glaser. Sept. 28, 1998. Stress-Associated Immune Modulation: Relevance to Viral Infections and Chronic Fatigue Syndrome. *Am J Med* 105(3A): 35S–42S.

Hässig, A., L. Wen-Xi, and K. Stampfli. June 1996. Stress-Induced Suppression of the Cellular Immune Reactions on the Neuroendocrine Control of the Immune System. *Med Hypotheses* 46(6): 551–55.

Mayr, B., and A. Mayr. July 1998. Interactions Between the Immune System and the Psyche. Lehrstuhl fur Mikrobiologie und Seuchenlehre, Tierarztlichen Fakultat, Ludwig-Maximihans-Universifat Munchen, *Tierarztl Prax Ausg K Klienfiere Heimtiere* 26(4):230–35.

Shephard, R. J., and P. N. Shek. 1998. Immunological Hazards from Nutritional Imbalance in Athletes. *Exerc Immunol Rev* 40: 22–48.

Venkatraman, J. T., et al. Mar. 1997. Influence of the Level of Dietary Lipid Intake and Maximal Exercise on the Immune Status in Runners. *Med Sci Sports Exerc* 29(3):333–44.

CHAPTER 20: THE OPTIMUM INTERFERON PROTOCOL

Davis, G. L., L. A. Balart, et al. Treatment of chronic hepatitis C with recombinant interferon alfa. A multicenter, randomized, controlled trial. *N Engl J Med* 1989; 321:1501–06.

Fried, M. W., M. L. Shiffman, R. Reddy, et al. Peginterferon alfa-2a plus ribavirin for chronic hepatitis C virus infection. *N Engl J Med* 2002; 347:975–82.

Hadziyannis, S. J., H. Sette Jr., T. R. Morgan, et al. Peginterferon alpha-2a and ribavirin combination therapy in chronic hepatitis C: a randomized study of treatment duration and ribavirin dose. *Ann Intern Med* 2004; 140:346–55.

Hauser P. Neuropsychiatric side effects of HCV therapy and their treatment: focus on IFN alpha-induced depression. *Gastroenterol Clin North Am* 2004; 33:S35–S50.

Hayasaka S., Y. Nagaki, M. Matsumoto, et al. Interferon associated retinopathy. *Br J Ophthalmol* 1998;82:323–325.

Hepatitis C Support Project. A Guide to Hepatitis C: Treatment Side Effect Management Vol. 1.0, www.HCVAdvocate.org October 2005.

Manns M. P., J. G. McHutchison, S. C. Gordon, et al. Peginterferon alfa-2b plus ribavirin compared with interferon alfa-2b plus ribavirin for initial treatment of chronic hepatitis C: a randomized trial. *Lancet* 2001; 358:958–65.

McHutchison J. G., S. C. Gordon, E. R. Schiff, et al. Interferon alfa-2b alone or in combination with ribavirin as initial treatment for chronic hepatitis C. *N Engl J Med* 1998; 339:1485–92.

Pegasys [package insert]. Nutley, N.J.: Hoffman-La Roche Inc.; December 2002.

Peg-Intron [package insert]. Kenilworth, N.J.: Schering Corporation; July 2002.

Torriani F. J., M. Rodriguez-Torres, J. K. Rockstroh, et al. Peginterferon alfa-2a plus ribavirin for chronic hepatitis C virus infection in HIV-infected patients. *N Engl J Med* 2004;351:438–50.

Index

About the Authors

MISHA RUTH COHEN, O.M.D., L.Ac.

Misha Ruth Cohen is an assistant researcher for Integrative Medicine at the University of California in San Francisco and research and education chair at Quan Yin Healing Arts Center. She is a pioneer and leader in North America in the use of Chinese traditional medicine for treating hepatitis C. Along with Dr. Gish, she is working in conjunction with some of the best Western researchers and clinicians in the hopes of forging a breakthrough treatment program. She frequently speaks to Western doctors and people with hepatitis C about the benefits of using Chinese traditional medicine as complementary therapy or alternative therapy for HCV, and she relays information to patients and physicians around the world on the East/West approach to HCV treatment. Through the Hepatitis C Professional Certification Program, she has trained more than two hundred Chinese medicine practitioners in how to treat people with HCV using Chinese medicine and natural approaches in conjunction with Western medicine. She estimates that in her private clinic, Chicken Soup Chinese Medicine, 50 to 60 percent of her clients are infected with HCV.

ROBERT G. GISH, M.D.

Robert G. Gish, M.D., is board certified in internal medicine and gastroenterology, a hepatologist and medical director of the Liver Disease Management and Transplant Program at the California Pacific Medical Center (CPMC) in San Francisco, as well as division chief of the section on hepatology and complex gastroenterology within the Physicians Foundation at CPMC. Dr. Gish is also an associate clinical professor of medicine at the University of Nevada in Reno, as well as the University of California, San Francisco. In addition, Dr. Gish has published more than two hundred original articles, reviews, abstracts, and book chapters regarding all aspects of liver disease and transplantation, and is a widely requested speaker both nationally and internationally.

KALIA DONER

Kalia Doner is the author or coauthor of twenty-five books on a wide range of subjects, including *The Chinese Way to Healing: Many Paths to Wholeness* and *The HIV Wellness Sourcebook* in collaboration with Misha Ruth Cohen, O.M.D., L.Ac. She is also editor-in-chief of *REMEDY* and of *Diabetes Focus* magazines.